NIST Special Publication 800-66 Revision 1

NIST
National Institute of
Standards and Technology
U.S. Department of Commerce

An Introductory Resource Guide for Implementing the Health Insurance Portability and Accountability Act (HIPAA) Security Rule

Matthew Scholl, Kevin Stine,
Joan Hash, Pauline Bowen, Arnold Johnson,
Carla Dancy Smith, and Daniel I. Steinberg

INFORMATION SECURITY

Computer Security Division
Information Technology Laboratory
National Institute of Standards and Technology
Gaithersburg, MD 20899-8930

October 2008

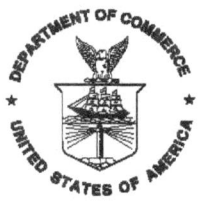

U.S. Department of Commerce
Carlos M. Gutierrez, Secretary
National Institute of Standards and Technology
Patrick D. Gallagher, Deputy Director

Reports on Information Systems Technology

The Information Technology Laboratory (ITL) at the National Institute of Standards and Technology (NIST) promotes the U.S. economy and public welfare by providing technical leadership for the nation's measurement and standards infrastructure. ITL develops tests, test methods, reference data, proof of concept implementations, and technical analyses to advance the development and productive use of information technology. ITL's responsibilities include the development of management, administrative, technical, and physical standards and guidelines for the cost-effective security and privacy of other than national security-related information in federal information systems. The Special Publication 800-series reports on ITL's research, guidelines, and outreach efforts in information system security, and its collaborative activities with industry, government, and academic organizations.

An Introductory Resource Guide for Implementing the Health Insurance Portability and Accountability Act (HIPAA) Security Rule

Authority

This document has been developed by the National Institute of Standards and Technology (NIST) to further its statutory responsibilities under the Federal Information Security Management Act (FISMA) of 2002, P.L. 107-347. NIST is responsible for developing standards and guidelines, including minimum requirements, for providing adequate information security for all agency operations and assets, but such standards and guidelines shall not apply to national security systems. This guideline is consistent with the requirements of the Office of Management and Budget (OMB) Circular A-130, Section 8b(3), Securing Agency Information Systems, as analyzed in A-130, Appendix IV: Analysis of Key Sections. Supplemental information is provided in A-130, Appendix III.

This guideline has been prepared for use by federal agencies. It may also be used by nongovernmental organizations on a voluntary basis and is not subject to copyright. (Attribution would be appreciated by NIST.)

Nothing in this document should be taken to contradict standards and guidelines made mandatory and binding on federal agencies by the Secretary of Commerce under statutory authority. Nor should these guidelines be interpreted as altering or superseding the existing authorities of the Secretary of Commerce, Director of the OMB, or any other federal official.

Certain commercial entities, equipment, or materials may be identified in this document in order to describe an experimental procedure or concept adequately. Such identification is not intended to imply recommendation or endorsement by the National Institute of Standards and Technology, nor is it intended to imply that the entities, materials, or equipment are necessarily the best available for the purpose.

There are references in this publication to documents currently under development by NIST in accordance with responsibilities assigned to NIST under the Federal Information Security Management Act of 2002. The methodologies in this document may be used even before the completion of such companion documents. Thus, until such time as each document is completed, current requirements, guidelines, and procedures (where they exist) remain operative. For planning and transition purposes, agencies may wish to closely follow the development of these new documents by NIST. Individuals are also encouraged to review the public draft documents and offer their comments to NIST. All NIST documents mentioned in this publication, other than the ones noted above, are available at http://csrc.nist.gov/publications.

Acknowledgments

The authors wish to thank their colleagues who helped update this document, prepared drafts, and reviewed materials. In addition, special thanks are due to Patricia Toth from NIST, and Lorraine Doo and Michael Phillips from the Centers for Medicare and Medicaid Services (CMS), who greatly contributed to the document's development. The authors also gratefully acknowledge and appreciate the many contributions from the public and private sectors whose thoughtful and constructive comments improved the quality and usefulness of this publication.

Disclaimer

This publication is intended as general guidance only for federal organizations, and is not intended to be, nor should it be construed or relied upon as legal advice or guidance to non federal entities or persons. This document does not modify the Health Insurance Portability and Accountability Act of 1996 (HIPAA) or any other federal law or regulation. The participation of other federal organizations with the National Institute of Standards and Technology (NIST) and NIST workgroups in the development of this special publication does not, and shall not be deemed to, constitute the endorsement, recommendation, or approval by those organizations of its contents.

Table of Contents

Executive Summary vii

1. Introduction 1
1.1. Purpose and Scope 2
1.2. Applicability 3
1.3. Audience 4
1.4. Document Organization 4
1.5. How and Why to Use This Document 5

2. Background 6
2.1. HIPAA Security Rule 6
2.1.1. Security Rule Goals and Objectives 6
2.1.2. Security Rule Organization 7
2.2. NIST and its Role in Information Security 9

3. A Framework for Managing Risk 10
3.1. NIST Risk Management Framework (RMF) 10
3.2. The NIST RMF and Links to the Security Rule 11

4. Considerations when Applying the HIPAA Security Rule 15

Administrative Safeguards 17
4.1. Security Management Process (§ 164.308(a)(1)) 17
4.2. Assigned Security Responsibility (§ 164.308(a)(2)) 20
4.3. Workforce Security (§ 164.308(a)(3)) 21
4.4. Information Access Management (§ 164.308(a)(4)) 23
4.5. Security Awareness and Training (§ 164.308(a)(5)) 25
4.6. Security Incident Procedures (§ 164.308(a)(6)) 27
4.7. Contingency Plan (§ 164.308(a)(7)) 29
4.8. Evaluation (§ 164.308(a)(8)) 31
4.9. Business Associate Contracts and Other Arrangements (§ 164.308(b)(1)). 33

Physical Safeguards 35
4.10. Facility Access Controls (§ 164.310(a)(1)) 35
4.11. Workstation Use (§ 164.310(b)) 37
4.12. Workstation Security (§ 164.310(c)) 38
4.13. Device and Media Controls (§ 164.310(d)(1)) 39

Technical Safeguards 40
4.14. Access Control (§ 164.312(a)(1)) 40
4.15. Audit Controls (§ 164.312(b)) 42
4.16. Integrity (§ 164.312(c)(1)) 44
4.17. Person or Entity Authentication (§ 164.312(d)) 46
4.18. Transmission Security (§ 164.312(e)(1)) 47

Organizational Requirements 48
   4.19.   Business Associate Contracts or Other Arrangements (§ 164.314(a)(1)) 48
   4.20.   Requirements for Group Health Plans (§ 164.314(b)(1)) 51

Policies and Procedures and Documentation Requirements 52
   4.21.   Policies and Procedures (§ 164.316(a)) 52
   4.22.   Documentation (§ 164.316(b)(1)) 53

Appendix A: Glossary A-1

Appendix B: Acronyms B-1

Appendix C: References C-1

Appendix D: Security Rule Standards and Implementation Specifications Crosswalk . D-1

Appendix E: Risk Assessment Guidelines E-1

Appendix F: Contingency Planning Guidelines F-1

Appendix G: Sample Contingency Plan Template G-1

Appendix H: Resources for Secure Remote Use and Access H-1

Appendix I: Telework Security Considerations I-1

Executive Summary

Some federal agencies, in addition to being subject to the Federal Information Security Management Act of 2002 (FISMA), are also subject to similar requirements of the Health Insurance Portability and Accountability Act of 1996 (HIPAA) Security Rule (the Security Rule), if the agency is a covered entity as defined by the rules implementing HIPAA.

The HIPAA Security Rule specifically focuses on the safeguarding of electronic protected health information (EPHI). Although FISMA applies to all federal agencies and all information types, only a subset of agencies are subject to the HIPAA Security Rule based on their functions and use of EPHI. All HIPAA covered entities, which include some federal agencies, must comply with the Security Rule, which specifically focuses on protecting the confidentiality, integrity, and availability of EPHI, as defined in the Security Rule. The EPHI that a covered entity creates, receives, maintains, or transmits must be protected against reasonably anticipated threats, hazards, and impermissible uses and/or disclosures. In general, the requirements, standards, and implementation specifications of the Security Rule apply to the following covered entities:

- Covered Healthcare Providers—Any provider of medical or other health services, or supplies, who transmits any health information in electronic form in connection with a transaction for which the Department of Health and Human Services (DHHS) has adopted a standard.

- Health Plans—Any individual or group plan that provides, or pays the cost of, medical care, including certain specifically listed governmental programs (e.g., a health insurance issuer and the Medicare and Medicaid programs).

- Healthcare Clearinghouses—A public or private entity that processes another entity's healthcare transactions from a standard format to a nonstandard format, or vice versa.

- Medicare Prescription Drug Card Sponsors—A nongovernmental entity that offered an endorsed discount drug program under the Medicare Modernization Act. This fourth category of "covered entity" remained in effect until the drug card program ended in 2006

NIST publications, many of which are required for federal agencies, can serve as voluntary guidelines and best practices for state, local, and tribal governments and the private sector, and may provide enough depth and breadth to help organizations of many sizes select the type of implementation that best fits their unique circumstances. NIST security standards and guidelines (Federal Information Processing Standards [FIPS], Special Publications in the 800 series), which can be used to support the requirements of both HIPAA and FISMA, may be used by organizations to help provide a structured, yet flexible framework for selecting, specifying, employing, and evaluating the security controls in information systems.

This Special Publication (SP), which discusses security considerations and resources that may provide value when implementing the requirements of the HIPAA Security Rule, was written to:

- Help to educate readers about information security terms used in the HIPAA Security Rule and to improve understanding of the meaning of the security standards set out in the Security Rule;

- Direct readers to helpful information in other NIST publications on individual topics addressed by the HIPAA Security Rule; and

- Aid readers in understanding the security concepts discussed in the HIPAA Security Rule. This publication does not supplement, replace, or supersede the HIPAA Security Rule itself.

1. Introduction

The National Institute of Standards and Technology (NIST) is responsible for developing standards and guidelines, including minimum requirements, used by federal agencies in providing adequate information security for the protection of agency operations and assets. Pursuant to this mission, NIST's Information Technology Laboratory (ITL) has developed guidelines to improve the efficiency and effectiveness of information technology (IT) planning, implementation, management, and operation.

NIST publishes a wide variety of publications on information security. These publications serve as a valuable resource for federal agencies, as well as public, nonfederal agencies and private organizations, seeking to address existing and new federal information security requirements. One such set of federal information security requirements are the security standards adopted by the Secretary of Health and Human Services (HHS) under the Health Insurance Portability and Accountability Act of 1996 (HIPAA, Public Law 104-191). HIPAA required the Secretary to adopt, among other standards, security standards for certain health information. These standards, known as the HIPAA Security Rule (the Security Rule), were published on February 20, 2003. In the preamble to the Security Rule, several NIST publications were cited as potentially valuable resources for readers with specific questions and concerns about IT security.

Congress enacted the Administrative Simplification (part of Title II) provisions of HIPAA to, among other things, promote efficiency in the healthcare industry through the use of standardized electronic transactions, while protecting the privacy and security of health information. Pursuant to the Administrative Simplification provisions of HIPAA, the Secretary of HHS adopted standards relating to:

- Electronic healthcare transactions and code sets;
- Privacy of protected health information;
- Security of electronic protected health information (EPHI); and
- Unique health identifiers.

This Special Publication summarizes the HIPAA security standards and explains some of the structure and organization of the Security Rule. The publication helps to educate readers about information security terms used in the HIPAA Security Rule and to improve understanding of the meaning of the security standards set out in the Security Rule. It is also designed to direct readers to helpful information in other NIST publications on individual topics addressed by the HIPAA Security Rule. Readers can draw upon these publications for consideration in implementing the Security Rule. This publication is intended as an aid to understanding security concepts discussed in the HIPAA Security Rule, and does not supplement, replace, or supersede the HIPAA Security Rule itself. While the Centers for Medicare and Medicaid Services (CMS) mentioned several NIST publications in the preamble to the HIPAA Security Rule, CMS does not require their use in complying with the Security Rule.[1]

---

[1] The HIPAA Security Rule mentions NIST documents as potentially helpful guidance but not mandatory for compliance, at 68 *Federal Register* pages 8346, 8350, 8352, and 8355 (February 20, 2003).

This document addresses only the security standards of the Security Rule and not other provisions adopted or raised by the Rule, such as 45 CFR § 164.105.

Figure 1 shows all the components of HIPAA and illustrates that the focus of this document is on the security provisions of the statute and the regulatory rule.

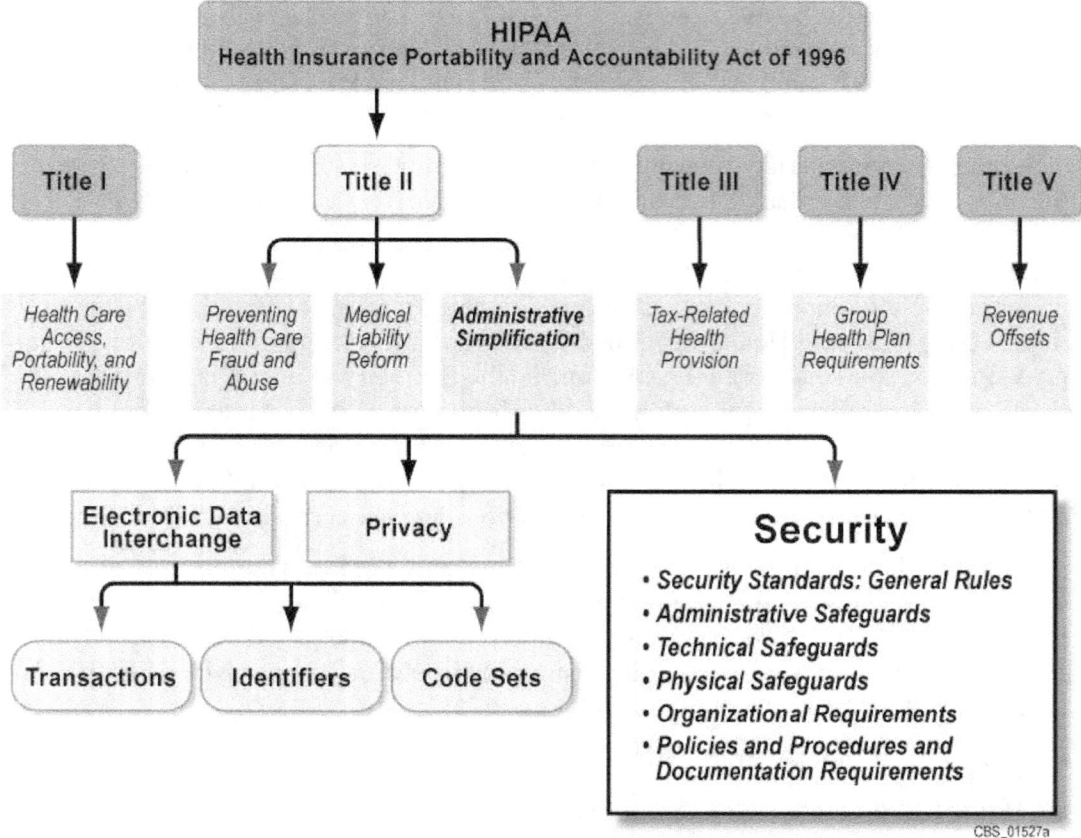

Figure 1. HIPAA Components

Readers should refer to the CMS Web site, http://www.cms.hhs.gov/HIPAAGenInfo/, for more detailed information about the passage of HIPAA by Congress, specific provisions of HIPAA, determination of the entities covered under the law, the complete text of the HIPAA Security Rule, the deadline for compliance with the Rule, and enforcement information.

1.1. Purpose and Scope

The purpose of this publication is to help educate readers about the security standards included in the HIPAA Security Rule. It provides a brief overview of the HIPAA Security Rule, directs the reader to additional NIST publications on information security, and identifies typical activities an agency should consider in implementing an information security program.

This publication is intended as an aid to understand security concepts discussed in the HIPAA Security Rule and does not supplement, replace, modify, or supersede the Security Rule itself. Anyone seeking clarifications of the HIPAA Security Rule should contact the Office of E-Health Standards and Services (OESS) at CMS. For general HIPAA Security Rule information, visit the CMS HIPAA Web site at: http://www.cms.hhs.gov/SecurityStandard/.

The NIST publications available as of the publication date of SP 800-66 Revision 1 were used in preparing this document. NIST frequently publishes new standards and guidelines, or updates existing publications that may also serve as useful references. To remain current with the latest available list of NIST security publications, the reader should periodically review the NIST Computer Security Resource Center (CSRC) Web site at http://csrc.nist.gov.

1.2. Applicability

The guidelines provided in this publication are applicable to all federal information systems,[2] other than those systems designated as national security systems as defined in 44 United States Code (U.S.C.), Section 3542.[3] The guidelines included in this publication have been broadly developed from a technical perspective so as to be complementary to similar guidelines issued by agencies and offices operating or exercising control over national security systems. State, local, and tribal governments, as well as private sector organizations composing the critical health infrastructure of the United States are encouraged to consider using these guidelines, as appropriate.

NIST publications may be useful to any agency seeking to understand the security issues raised by the HIPAA Security Rule regardless of that agency's size, structure, or distribution of security responsibilities. Specific agency missions, resources, and organizational structures, however, vary greatly, and agencies' approaches to implementing the HIPAA Security Rule may diverge significantly. Federal agencies use different titles to identify roles that have security-related responsibilities and may also assign particular responsibilities for implementing information security controls (those required by HIPAA and others) differently. NIST SP 800-66 assists all agencies seeking further information on the security safeguards discussed in the HIPAA Security Rule, regardless of the particular structures, methodologies, and approaches used to address its requirements.

---

[2] A federal information system is an information system used or operated by an executive agency, by a contractor of an executive agency, or by another organization on behalf of an executive agency.

[3] A national security system is any information system (including any telecommunications system) used or operated by an agency or by a contractor of an agency, or other organization on behalf of an agency—(i) the function, operation, or use of which: involves intelligence activities, involves cryptographic activities related to national security; involves command and control of military forces; involves equipment that is an integral part of a weapon or weapons system; or is critical to the direct fulfillment of military or intelligence missions (excluding a system that is to be used for routine administrative and business applications, for example, payroll, finance, logistics, and personnel management applications); or (ii) is protected at all times by procedures established for information that have been specifically authorized under criteria established by an Executive Order or an Act of Congress to be kept classified in the interest of national defense or foreign policy. Agencies should consult NIST Special Publication 800-59, *Guide for Identifying an Information System as a National Security System*, for guidance on determining the status of their information systems.

The preamble of the Security Rule states that HHS does not rate or endorse the use of industry-developed guidelines and/or models. Organizations that are not required to use this NIST special publication (by other regulation, law, or requirement) yet choose to use it, must determine the value of its content for implementing the Security Rule standards in their environments. The use of this publication or any other NIST publication does not ensure or guarantee that an organization will be compliant with the Security Rule.

1.3. Audience

This publication is intended to serve a diverse audience of individuals with HIPAA Security Rule implementation, management, and oversight responsibilities and organizations, federal and nonfederal, considered to be a "Covered Entity" under 45 C.F.R. Sec.160.103.

1.4. Document Organization

The remaining sections and appendices of this publication include the following:

Section 2 - Background explains the key concepts included in the HIPAA Security Rule and provides an overview of NIST's role in information security, as well as descriptions of its various information security publications.

Section 3 – Risk Management Framework introduces a structured, flexible, extensible, and repeatable process for managing organizational risk and achieving risk-based protection related to the operation and use of information systems, and the protection of EPHI.

Section 4 – Considerations When Applying the HIPAA Security Rule highlights key activities a covered entity may wish to consider when implementing the Security Rule.

Appendix A – Glossary defines terms used in this document.

Appendix B – Acronyms identifies and defines acronyms used within this document.

Appendix C – References provides references and related source material.

Appendix D – Security Rule Standards and Implementation Specifications Crosswalk provides a catalog of the HIPAA Security Rule standards and implementation specifications, and crosswalks each to relevant NIST publications and security controls detailed in NIST SP 800-53, *Recommended Security Controls for Federal Information Systems*.

Appendix E – Risk Assessment Guidelines provides a methodology for conducting a risk assessment, the results of which will enable covered entities to identify appropriate security controls for reducing risk to the organization and its data and information systems.

Appendix F – Contingency Planning Guidelines identifies fundamental planning principles and practices to help covered entities develop and maintain effective information system contingency plans.

Appendix G – Sample Contingency Plan Template provides a template for preparing an information technology (IT) contingency plan.

Appendix H – Resources for Secure Remote Use and Access provides an overview of NIST publications discussing security technologies that may provide value for organizations facing challenges in securing remotely accessible, stored, or transmitted EPHI.

Appendix I – Telework Security Considerations provides considerations and tips for securing external devices used for telework and remote access.

1.5. How and Why to Use This Document

Users are encouraged to use this document as a resource that provides concepts and tools to assist covered entities, including federal agencies, to comply with the HIPAA Security Rule.

NIST publications, many of which are required for federal agencies, can serve as guidelines and best practices for state, local, and tribal governments, and the private sector, and may provide enough depth and breadth to help organizations of many sizes select the type of implementation that best fits their unique circumstances.

This document can support the compliance efforts of covered entities in many ways, including:

- Ensuring that each organization is selecting methods and controls which adequately and appropriately protect EPHI of which they are the steward;

- Informing the development of compliance strategies that are in concert with the size and structure of the entity;

- Providing guidelines on best practices for developing and implementing a Risk Management Program; and

- Creating appropriate documentation that demonstrates effective compliance with the HIPAA Security Rule.

2. Background

2.1. HIPAA Security Rule

The HIPAA Security Rule specifically focuses on the safeguarding of EPHI. Although FISMA applies to all federal agencies and all information types, only a subset of agencies is subject to the HIPAA Security Rule based on their functions and use of EPHI. All HIPAA covered entities, which includes some federal agencies, must comply with the Security Rule. The Security Rule specifically focuses on protecting the confidentiality, integrity, and availability of EPHI, as defined in the Security Rule. The EPHI that a covered entity creates, receives, maintains, or transmits must be protected against reasonably anticipated threats, hazards, and impermissible uses and/or disclosures. In general, the requirements, standards, and implementation specifications of the Security Rule apply to the following covered entities:

- **Covered Healthcare Providers**— Any provider of medical or other health services, or supplies, who transmits any health information in electronic form in connection with a transaction for which HHS has adopted a standard.

- **Health Plans**— Any individual or group plan that provides or pays the cost of medical care (e.g., a health insurance issuer and the Medicare and Medicaid programs).

- **Healthcare Clearinghouses**— A public or private entity that processes another entity's healthcare transactions from a standard format to a nonstandard format, or vice versa.

- **Medicare Prescription Drug Card Sponsors** – A nongovernmental entity that offers an endorsed discount drug program under the Medicare Modernization Act.

This section identifies the main goals, explains some of the structure and organization, and identifies the purpose of the sections of the Security Rule.

2.1.1. Security Rule Goals and Objectives

As required by the "Security standards: General rules"[4] section of the HIPAA Security Rule, each covered entity must:

- Ensure the confidentiality, integrity, and availability of EPHI that it creates, receives, maintains, or transmits;

- Protect against any reasonably anticipated threats and hazards to the security or integrity of EPHI; and

- Protect against reasonably anticipated uses or disclosures of such information that are not permitted by the Privacy Rule.

---

[4] See 45 C.F.R. § 164.306(a).

In complying with this section of the Security Rule, covered entities must be aware of the definitions provided for confidentiality, integrity, and availability as given by § 164.304:

- **Confidentiality** is "the property that data or information is not made available or disclosed to unauthorized persons or processes."
- **Integrity** is "the property that data or information have not been altered or destroyed in an unauthorized manner."
- **Availability** is "the property that data or information is accessible and useable upon demand by an authorized person."

2.1.2. Security Rule Organization

To understand the requirements of the HIPAA Security Rule, it is helpful to be familiar with the basic security terminology it uses to describe the security standards. By understanding the requirements and the terminology in the HIPAA Security Rule, it becomes easier to see which NIST publications may be appropriate reference resources and where to find more information. The Security Rule is separated into six main sections that each include several standards and implementation specifications that a covered entity must address.[5] The six sections are listed below.

- **Security standards: General Rules** - includes the general requirements all covered entities must meet; establishes flexibility of approach; identifies standards and implementation specifications (both required and addressable); outlines decisions a covered entity must make regarding addressable implementation specifications; and requires maintenance of security measures to continue reasonable and appropriate protection of electronic protected health information.

- **Administrative Safeguards** - are defined in the Security Rule as the "administrative actions and policies, and procedures to manage the selection, development, implementation, and maintenance of security measures to protect electronic protected health information and to manage the conduct of the covered entity's workforce in relation to the protection of that information."

- **Physical Safeguards** - are defined as the "physical measures, policies, and procedures to protect a covered entity's electronic information systems and related buildings and equipment, from natural and environmental hazards, and unauthorized intrusion."

- **Technical Safeguards** - are defined as the "the technology and the policy and procedures for its use that protect electronic protected health information and control access to it."

---

[5] Sections of the HIPAA regulations that are included in the Security Rule and therefore addressed in this document but do not have their own modules are *Part 160 — General Administrative Requirements* § 160.103, *Definitions*; *Part 164 — Security and Privacy* §§ 164.103, *Definitions*; 164.104, *Applicability*, 164.105, *Organizational requirements* (discussed in section 4 of this document), 164.302 *Applicability*, 164.304, *Definitions*; 164.306, *Security standards: General rules* (discussed in section 3 of this document), and 164.318, *Compliance dates for the initial implementation of the security standards.*

- **Organizational Requirements** - includes standards for business associate contracts and other arrangements, including memoranda of understanding between a covered entity and a business associate when both entities are government organizations; and requirements for group health plans.

- **Policies and Procedures and Documentation Requirements** - requires implementation of reasonable and appropriate policies and procedures to comply with the standards, implementation specifications and other requirements of the Security Rule; maintenance of written (which may be electronic) documentation and/or records that includes policies, procedures, actions, activities, or assessments required by the Security Rule; and retention, availability, and update requirements related to the documentation.

Within the Security Rule sections are standards and implementation specifications. Each HIPAA Security Rule standard is required. A covered entity is required to comply with all standards of the Security Rule with respect to all EPHI.

Many of the standards contain implementation specifications. An implementation specification is a more detailed description of the method or approach covered entities can use to meet a particular standard.[6] Implementation specifications are either required or addressable. However, regardless of whether a standard includes implementation specifications, covered entities must comply with each standard.

- A **required** implementation specification is similar to a standard, in that a covered entity must comply with it.

- For **addressable** implementation specifications, covered entities must perform an assessment to determine whether the implementation specification is a reasonable and appropriate safeguard for implementation in the covered entity's environment. In general, after performing the assessment, a covered entity decides if it will implement the addressable implementation specification; implement an equivalent alternative measure that allows the entity to comply with the standard; or not implement the addressable specification or any alternative measures, if equivalent measures are not reasonable and appropriate within its environment. Covered entities are required to document these assessments and all decisions. For federal agencies, however, all of the HIPAA Security Rule's addressable implementation specifications will most likely be reasonable and appropriate safeguards for implementation, given their sizes, missions, and resources.

Where there are no implementation specifications identified in the Security Rule for a particular standard, such as for the "Assigned Security Responsibility" and "Evaluation" standards, compliance with the standard itself is required.

Appendix D of this document provides a crosswalk of the HIPAA Security Rule standards and implementation specifications to relevant NIST publications and security controls detailed in NIST SP 800-53.

---

[6] For more information on the required analysis used to determine the manner of implementation of an implementation specification, see § 164.306(d) of the HIPAA Security Rule (Security standards — General rules: Flexibility of approach).

For general HIPAA Security Rule information, visit the CMS HIPAA Web site at http://www.cms.hhs.gov/SecurityStandard/.

2.2. NIST and its Role in Information Security

Founded in 1901, NIST is a non-regulatory federal agency within the U.S. Department of Commerce. NIST's mission is to promote U.S. innovation and industrial competitiveness by advancing measurement science, standards, and technology in ways that enhance economic security and improve our quality of life. NIST is composed of several laboratories that conduct research in a wide variety of physical and engineering sciences. Lab researchers respond to industry needs for measurement methods, tools, data, and technology, and collaborate with colleagues in industry, academic institutions, and other government agencies.

The Computer Security Division (CSD), a component within NIST's Information Technology Laboratory (ITL), provides standards and technology to protect information systems against threats to the confidentiality of information, the integrity of information and processes, and the availability of information and services in order to build trust and confidence in IT systems.

CSD develops and issues standards, guidelines, and other publications to assist federal agencies in implementing the requirements of FISMA and in managing cost-effective security programs to protect their information and information systems. Table 1 identifies and describes the types of NIST publications.

Table 1: NIST Publication Types

Publication Type	Description
Federal Information Processing Standards (FIPS)	Developed by NIST in accordance with FISMA. They are approved by the Secretary of Commerce and are compulsory and binding for federal agencies. Since FISMA requires that federal agencies comply with these standards, agencies may not waive their use. FIPS may be used voluntarily by nonfederal organizations (e.g., state/local/tribal governments, industry).
Special Publication (SP) 800-series	Reports on ITL's research, guidelines, and outreach efforts in information system security and its collaborative activities with industry, government, and academia. Office of Management and Budget (OMB) policies state that for other than national security programs and systems, federal agencies must follow NIST guidelines. SPs may be used voluntarily by nonfederal organizations.
Other Security Publications	Other publications including interagency reports (NISTIRs) and ITL bulletins that provide technical and other information about NIST's activities.

3. A Framework for Managing Risk

The HIPAA Security Rule is all about implementing effective risk management to adequately and effectively protect EPHI. The assessment, analysis, and management of risk provides the foundation of a covered entity's Security Rule compliance efforts, serving as tools to develop and maintain a covered entity's strategy to protect the confidentiality, integrity, and availability of EPHI.

All EPHI created, received, maintained, or transmitted by a covered entity is subject to the Security Rule. Covered entities are required to implement reasonable and appropriate security measures to protect against reasonably anticipated threats or vulnerabilities to the security of EPHI. Under the Security Rule, covered entities are required to evaluate risks and vulnerabilities in their environments and to implement security controls to address those risks and vulnerabilities.

The selection and specification of security controls can be accomplished as part of an organization-wide information security program that involves the management of organizational risk - that is, the risk to information, individuals, and the organization as a whole. The management of risk is a key element in the organization's information security program and provides an effective framework for selecting the appropriate security controls for an information system - the security controls necessary to protect individuals and the operations and assets of the organization.

This section describes a process of managing risk to organizational missions and business functions that arise from the operation and use of information systems by discussing each phase of the NIST Risk Management Framework[7] and providing a mapping of this framework to complementary requirements of the HIPAA Security Rule.

3.1. NIST Risk Management Framework (RMF)

The NIST RMF, illustrated in Figure 2, provides the covered entity with a disciplined, structured, extensible, and repeatable process for achieving risk-based protection related to the operation and use of information systems and the protection of EPHI. It represents an information security life cycle that facilitates continuous monitoring and improvement in the security state of the information systems within the organization.

The activities that compose the NIST RMF are paramount to an effective information security program and can be applied to both new and legacy information systems within the context of a system development life cycle. A risk-based approach to security control selection and specification considers effectiveness, efficiency, and constraints due to applicable laws, directives, Executive Orders, policies, standards, or regulations.

The flexible nature of the NIST RMF allows other communities of interest (e.g., state, local, and tribal governments and private sector entities) to use the framework voluntarily either with the NIST security standards and guidelines or with industry-specific standards and guidelines. The RMF provides organizations with the flexibility needed to apply the right security controls to the right information systems at the right time to adequately

---

[7] NIST Special Publication 800-39, *Managing Risk from Information Systems: An Organizational Perspective*, (Second Public Draft), April 2008.

protect the critical and sensitive information, missions, and business functions of the organization.

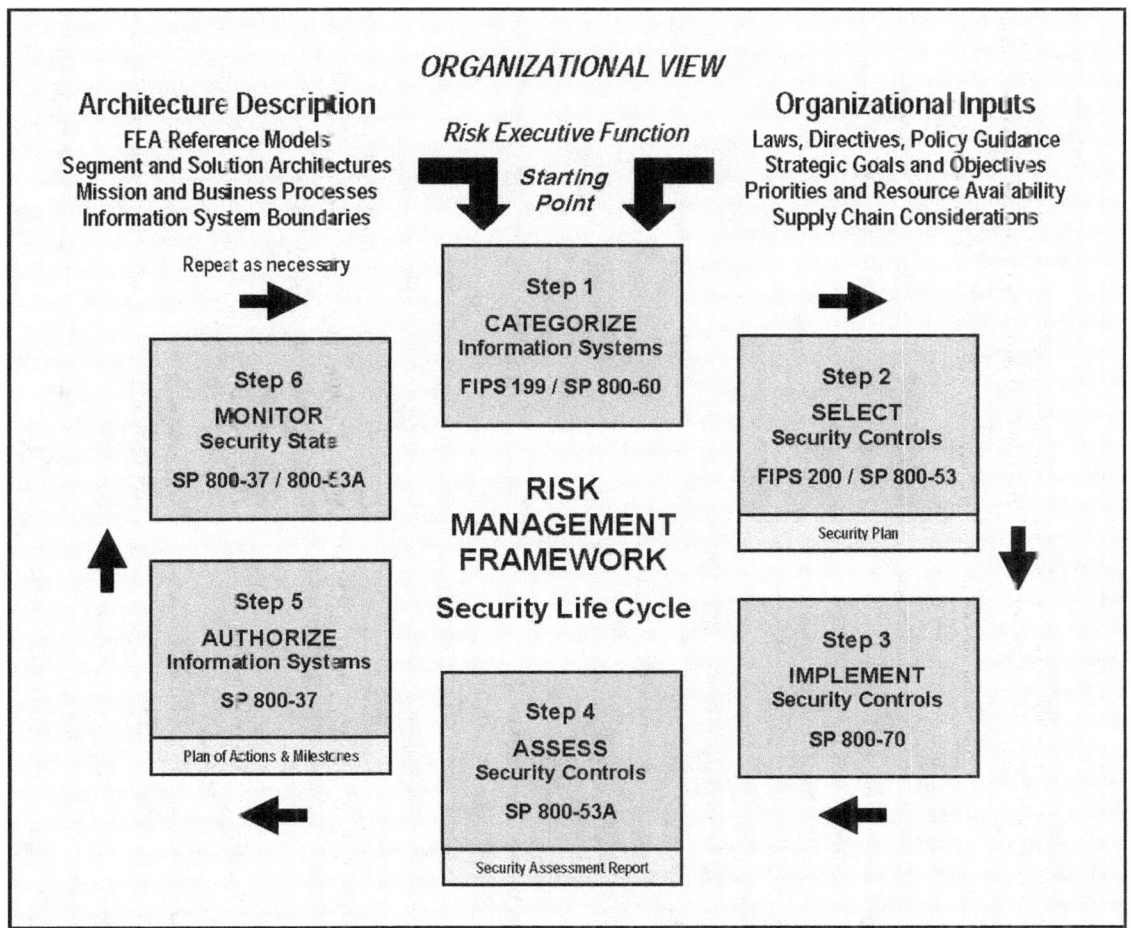

Figure 2. NIST Risk Management Framework

3.2. The NIST RMF and Links to the Security Rule

The NIST RMF consists of six steps that are paramount to the effective management of risk resulting from the operation and use of information systems. Many Security Rule standards and implementation specifications correspond to the steps of the NIST RMF. Using these corresponding requirements in an integrated fashion can provide a methodical, repeatable, risk-based approach for selecting, specifying, and implementing security controls to adequately protect EPHI. Table 2 describes each step in the NIST RMF as well as the related standards and implementation specifications found in the Security Rule.

Table 2: Linking the NIST RMF and the Security Rule

RMF Phase	RMF Step Description	Security Rule Link
Categorize Information Systems	Security categorization, the first and arguably the most important step in the RMF, employs FIPS 199 and NIST SP 800-60 to determine the criticality and sensitivity of the information system and the information being processed, stored, and transmitted by the system. This exercise aids in determining priorities for organizational information systems and subsequently applying appropriate measures to adequately protect the organizational missions and business functions supported by those missions. The security controls applied to a particular information system should be commensurate with the potential impact on organizational operations and assets, individuals, or other organizations should there be a loss of confidentiality, integrity, or availability.	Identify assets and information systems that create, receive, transmit, or maintain EPHI. *Related Standards and Implementation Specifications:* 164.308(a)(1)(i) – Security Management Process
Select Security Controls	Security control selection, the second step in the RMF, employs FIPS 200 and NIST SP 800-53 to identify and specify appropriate security controls for the information system. The selection of security controls for an organization's mission/business processes and the information systems supporting those processes is a risk mitigation activity. The security control selection process consists of three activities: • Selection of baseline security controls for each information system from NIST SP 800-53 in accordance with FIPS 199 impact levels determined during the security categorization process; • Application of security control tailoring guidance for the information systems to allow organizations to adjust the initial security control baselines with respect to specific mission and business processes,	Select the standards and required implementation specifications as the initial security control set. These required security controls establish the baseline from which to assess risk to EPHI. Once the baseline is established, perform a risk assessment and analysis to evaluate whether the standards and required implementation specifications alone are reasonable and appropriate to provide adequate protection against reasonably anticipated threats or hazards to the confidentiality, integrity, or availability of EPHI. The results of this risk assessment and analysis will drive the selection of addressable implementation specifications to adequately supplement the baseline. Supplement the initial set of standards and required implementation specifications (baseline) with addressable implementation specifications. The decisions to supplement

RMF Phase	RMF Step Description	Security Rule Link
	organizational requirements, and environments of operations; and • Supplementation of tailored baseline security controls with additional controls based on an assessment of risk and local conditions including specific and credible threat information, organization-specific security requirements, cost-benefit analyses, and special circumstances. Key to this process is documenting the selection and specification of security controls. A documented security plan provides an overview of the security requirements for the information systems within the organization and describes the security controls in place or planned for meeting those requirements. Additionally, the security plans for organizational information systems describe how individual security controls are implemented within specific operational environments. It is important for organizations to document the decisions taken during the security control selection process, providing a sound rationale for those decisions. The resulting set of security controls along with the supporting rationale for security control selection decisions and any information system use restrictions are documented in the security plans for the information system. This provides a clear description of the risk mitigation deemed necessary in order to adequately ensure mission accomplishment and success of business functions potentially impacted by the operation and use of the systems.	the security control baseline should be based on an assessment of risk and local conditions including organization-specific security requirements, specific threat information, cost-benefit analyses, or special circumstances. The agreed-upon set of security controls will consist of the standards, required implementation specifications, and the risk-based selection of addressable implementation specifications. Each covered entity must document the security controls determined to be reasonable and appropriate, including analysis, decisions, and rationale for decisions made to refine or adjust the security controls *Related Standards and Implementation Specifications:* 164.308(a)(1)(i) – Security Management Process 164.308(a)(1)(ii)(A) – Risk Analysis 164.308(a)(1)(ii)(B) – Risk Management 164.316(b)(1) – Documentation 164.316(b)(2)(ii) – Updates
Implement Security Controls	Security control implementation, the third step in the RMF, employs enterprise architectures, the System Development Lifecycle (SDLC), and various NIST publications to guide the implementation of security controls in organizational information systems.	Implement the security controls that have been determined to be reasonable and appropriate for the organization. *Related Standards and Implementation Specifications:* 164.308(a)(1)(ii)(B) – Risk Management

RMF Phase	RMF Step Description	Security Rule Link
Assess Security Controls	Security Controls Assessment, the fourth step in the RMF, employs NIST SP 800-53A to evaluate the information system security controls for effectiveness using appropriate methods and procedures to determine the extent to which the controls are implemented correctly, operating as intended, and producing the desired outcome with respect to meeting the security objectives and requirements for the system.	Evaluate the implemented specifications using assessment methods and procedures to determine the extent to which the controls are implemented correctly and operating as intended with respect to protecting EPHI. *Related Standards and Implementation Specifications:* 164.308(a)(8) – Evaluation
Authorize Information System	Authorize information system operation (with implemented security controls) based upon a determination of the risk to organizational operations, organizational assets, individuals, and other organizations, and an explicit decision to accept this risk.	Inherent in any risk management process is the acceptance of those identified risks that are deemed acceptable to the organization. *Related Standards and Implementation Specifications:* 164.308(a)(1)(ii)(B) – Risk Management
Monitor Security State	Threats and vulnerabilities to an operating environment, as well as safeguards designed to combat them, can change frequently. The assessment and evaluation of security controls on a continuous basis provides oversight and monitoring of the security controls to ensure that they continue to operate effectively and as intended. Monitor and assess selected security controls in the information system on a continuous basis including documenting changes to the system, conducting security impact analyses of the changes, and reporting the system security status to appropriate organizational officials on a regular basis.	A covered entity must periodically review and update its security measures and documentation in response to environmental and operational changes that affect security of its EPHI. *Related Standards and Implementation Specifications:* 164.308(a)(8) – Evaluation 164.308(a)(1)(ii)(D) – Information System Activity Review

4. Considerations when Applying the HIPAA Security Rule

In this section, security measures from NIST publications that are relevant to each section of the Security Rule are presented. Each standard is presented in a consistent tabular format.

The following tables, organized by HIPAA Security Rule standard, are designed to initiate the thought process for implementing the requirements of the Security Rule. These tables highlight information a covered entity may wish to consider when implementing the Security Rule; they are not meant to be prescriptive. The tables may also not be considered all-inclusive of the information available in NIST publications.

In addition to the HIPAA Security Rule standard name and description, each table includes the following information:

- **Key Activities** - The Key Activities column suggests, for each HIPAA Security Rule standard, actions that are usually associated with the security function or functions suggested by that standard. Some of these key activities are also the implementation specifications for that particular standard. Each key activity that is also an implementation specification has been identified as such in the table (in italics in the Description section of the table), along with a note as to whether the implementation specification is required or addressable. Other key activities would normally be performed as part of one or more of the related implementation specifications under the standard, but are listed separately for clarity of presentation. Where such a relationship exists, it is indicated in an accompanying footnote.

Other key activities are not implementation specifications. These activities are not specifically discussed or required by the HIPAA Security Rule, and their inclusion here is in no way meant to expand upon the intent or requirements of the Security Rule. Many of these activities, however, are usually included in a robust security process, and many will be required of federal entities under other federal laws, regulations, or procedures that may or may not be discussed within this document.

The tables address all HIPAA Security Rule standards and all associated implementation specifications, both required and addressable. Seven of the standards include all the necessary instructions for implementation and have no associated implementation specifications.[8] However, as noted earlier in this document, even if there are no implementation specifications outlined in the Security Rule, such as with *Assigned Security Responsibility* and *Evaluation*, compliance with the standard itself is still required.

The key activities are illustrative and not all-inclusive. There may be many additional activities an organization will need to consider, specific to its own operations, which are not included in the key activities of the tables. Each entity will need to identify what activities beyond those listed in the tables are necessary and appropriate in its environment, implement those activities, and document them.

---

[8] Standards that do not contain implementation specifications—that "themselves also serve as the implementation specification," as stated in the preamble to the HIPAA Security Rule—are those described in Sections 4.2 (*HIPAA Standard: Assigned Security Responsibility*); 4.8 (*HIPAA Standard: Evaluation*); 4.11 (*HIPAA Standard: Workstation Use*); 4.12 (*HIPAA Standard: Workstation Security*), 4.15 (*HIPAA Standard: Audit Controls*); 4.17 (*HIPAA Standard: Person or Entity Authentication*); and 4.21 (*HIPAA Standard: Policies and Procedures*).

The tables are meant to serve as only a general introduction to the security topics raised by the HIPAA Security Rule. For more detailed information about the key activities, consult one or more NIST publications referenced for the subject HIPAA standard.

- **Description** - The Description column in each table includes an expanded explanation about the key activities. The descriptions include types of activities an organization may pursue in addressing a specific security function. These are abbreviated explanations designed to help get an organization started in addressing the HIPAA Security Rule. The first description bullet of each key activity that is also an implementation specification includes the Security Rule implementation specification text in italics. When relationships exist between description bullets and other Security Rule standards or implementation specifications, it is indicated in an accompanying footnote.

- **Sample Questions** - The Sample Questions column includes some questions to determine whether or not the elements described have actually been considered or completed. These sample questions are not exhaustive but merely indicative of relevant questions that could be asked. Affirmative answers to these questions do not imply that an organization is meeting all of the requirements of the HIPAA security standards. Negative answers to these questions should prompt the covered entity to consider whether it needs to take further action in order to comply with the standards. In fact, it is expected that many organizations with existing information security infrastructure already in place will have considered most of the Sample Questions. The questions an organization asks in assessing and developing its security program should be tailored to fit the unique circumstances of each entity.

This document does not discuss Section 164.105 of the HIPAA Security Rule, *Organizational Requirements,* in detail as they do not set out general security principles. HIPAA covered entities are encouraged to review this section of the HIPAA Security Rule in full and seek further guidance.

Administrative Safeguards

4.1. Security Management Process (§ 164.308(a)(1))

HIPAA Standard: *Implement policies and procedures to prevent, detect, contain, and correct security violations.*

Key Activities	Description	Sample Questions
1. Identify Relevant Information Systems	• Identify all information systems that house EPHI. • Include all hardware and software that are used to collect, store, process, or transmit EPHI. • Analyze business functions and verify ownership and control of information system elements as necessary.	• Are all hardware and software for which the organization is responsible periodically inventoried? • Have hardware and software that maintains or transmits EPHI been identified? Does this inventory include removable media and remote access devices? • Is the current information system configuration documented, including connections to other systems? • Have the types of information and uses of that information been identified and the sensitivity of each type of information been evaluated? (See FIPS 199 and SP 800-60 for more on categorization of sensitivity levels.)
2. Conduct Risk Assessment[9] Implementation Specification (Required)	*Conduct an accurate and thorough assessment of the potential risks and vulnerabilities to the confidentiality, integrity, and availability of EPHI held by the covered entity.* A risk assessment methodology, based on NIST SP 800-30, is included in Appendix E of this document.	• Are there any prior risk assessments, audit comments, security requirements, and/or security test results? • Is there intelligence available from agencies, the Office of the Inspector General (OIG), the US-CERT, virus alerts, and/or vendors? • What are the current and planned controls? • Is the facility located in a region prone to any natural disasters, such as earthquakes, floods, or fires? • Has responsibility been assigned to check all hardware and software, including hardware and software used for remote access, to determine whether selected security settings are enabled? • Is there an analysis of current safeguards and their effectiveness relative to the identified risks? • Have all processes involving EPHI been considered, including creating, receiving, maintaining, and transmitting it?
3. Implement a Risk Management Program[10]	*Implement security measures sufficient to reduce risks and vulnerabilities to a reasonable and appropriate level to comply with §164.306(a).*	• Do current safeguards ensure the confidentiality, integrity, and availability of all EPHI? • Do current safeguards protect against reasonably

---

[9] The risks that must be assessed are the risks of noncompliance with the requirements of Section 164.306(a) (General Rules) of the HIPAA Security Rule.
[10] See Section 164.306 of the HIPAA Security Rule.

An Introductory Resource Guide for Implementing the Health Insurance Portability and Accountability Act (HIPAA) Security Rule

Key Activities	Description	Sample Questions
Implementation Specification (Required)		• anticipated uses or disclosures of EPHI that are not permitted by the Privacy Rule? • Has the covered entity protected against all reasonably anticipated threats or hazards to the security and integrity of EPHI? • Has the covered entity assured compliance with all policies and procedures by its workforce?

4. Acquire IT Systems and Services[11, 12]	• Although the HIPAA Security Rule does not require purchasing any particular technology, additional hardware, software, or services may be needed to adequately protect information. Considerations for their selection should include the following:
	  ○ Applicability of the IT solution to the intended environment;
	  ○ The sensitivity of the data;
	  ○ The organization's security policies, procedures, and standards; and
	  ○ Other requirements such as resources available for operation, maintenance, and training.
		• Will new security controls work with the existing IT architecture?
		• Have the security requirements of the organization been compared with the security features of existing or proposed hardware and software?
		• Has a cost-benefit analysis been conducted to determine the reasonableness of the investment given the security risks identified?
		• Has a training strategy been developed?[13]

5. Create and Deploy Policies and Procedures[14, 15]	• Implement the decisions concerning the management, operational, and technical controls selected to mitigate identified risks. • Create policies that clearly establish roles and responsibilities and assign ultimate responsibility for the implementation of each control to particular individuals or offices.[16] • Create procedures to be followed to accomplish particular security-related tasks.	• Are policies and procedures in place for security? • Is there a formal (documented) system security plan? • Is there a formal contingency plan?[17] • Is there a process for communicating policies and procedures to the affected employees? • Are policies and procedures reviewed and updated as needed?
6. Develop and Implement a Sanction Policy[18] Implementation Specification (Required)	• Apply appropriate sanctions against workforce members who fail to comply with the security policies and procedures of the covered entity. • Develop policies and procedures for imposing appropriate sanctions (e.g., reprimand, termination) for noncompliance with the organization's security policies. • Implement sanction policy as cases arise.	• Is there a formal process in place to address system misuse, abuse, and fraudulent activity? • Have employees been made aware of policies concerning sanctions for inappropriate access, use, and disclosure of EPHI? • Has the need and appropriateness of a tiered structure of sanctions that accounts for the magnitude of harm and

[11] See Section 164.306(b) of the HIPAA Security Rule.
[12] See Key Activity 4.1.3, *Implement a Risk Management Program*. This activity and all associated bullets in the Description and Sample Questions are part of the process of addressing the risk management implementation specification.
[13] See Section 4.5, *HIPAA Standard: Security Awareness and Training*.
[14] See Section 4.21, *HIPAA Standard: Policies and Procedures*.
[15] See Key Activity 4.1.3, *Implement a Risk Management Program*. This activity and all associated bullets in the Description and Sample Questions are part of the process of addressing the risk management implementation specification.
[16] See Section 4.21, *HIPAA Standard: Policies and Procedures* and Section 4.22, *HIPAA Standard: Documentation*.
[17] See Section 4.7, *HIPAA Standard: Contingency Plan*.

An Introductory Resource Guide for Implementing the Health Insurance Portability and Accountability Act (HIPAA) Security Rule

Key Activities	Description	Sample Questions
		possible types of inappropriate disclosures been considered? • How will managers and employees be notified regarding suspect activity?
7. **Develop and Deploy the Information System Activity Review Process** Implementation Specification (Required)	• *Implement procedures to regularly review records of information system activity, such as audit logs, access reports, and security incident tracking reports.*	• Who is responsible for the overall process and results?[19] • How often will reviews take place? • How often will review results be analyzed? • What is the organization's sanction policy for employee violations? • Where will audit information reside (e.g., separate server)?
8. **Develop Appropriate Standard Operating Procedures**[20]	• Determine the types of audit trail data and monitoring procedures that will be needed to derive exception reports.	• How will exception reports or logs be reviewed? • Where will monitoring reports be filed and maintained?
9. **Implement the Information System Activity Review and Audit Process**[21]	• Activate the necessary review process. • Begin auditing and logging activity.	• What mechanisms will be implemented to assess the effectiveness of the review process (measures)? • What is the plan to revise the review process when needed?

---

[18] See Section 164.306 of the HIPAA Security Rule.
[19] See Section 4.2, *HIPAA Standard: Assigned Security Responsibility.*
[20] See Key Activity 4.1.7, *Develop and Deploy the Information System Activity Review Process.* This activity and all associated bullets in the Description and Sample Questions are part of the process of addressing the information system activity review implementation specification.
[21] See Key Activity 4.1.7, *Develop and Deploy the Information System Activity Review Process.* This activity and all associated bullets in the Description and Sample Questions are part of the process of addressing the information system activity review implementation specification.

4.2. Assigned Security Responsibility (§ 164.308(a)(2))

HIPAA Standard: *Identify the security official who is responsible for the development and implementation of the policies and procedures required by this subpart for the entity.*

Key Activities	Description	Sample Questions
1. Select a Security Official To Be Assigned Responsibility for HIPAA Security	<ul><li>Identify the individual who has final responsibility for security.</li><li>Select an individual who is able to assess effective security and to serve as the point of contact for security policy, implementation, and monitoring.</li></ul>	<ul><li>Who in the organization—<ul><li>Oversees the development and communication of security policies and procedures?</li><li>Is responsible for conducting the risk assessment?</li><li>Handles the results of periodic security evaluations and continuous monitoring?</li><li>Directs IT security purchasing and investment?</li><li>Ensures that security concerns have been addressed in system implementation?</li></ul></li><li>Who in the organization is authorized to accept risk from information systems on behalf of the organization?</li></ul>
2. Assign and Document the Individual's Responsibility	<ul><li>Document the assignment to one individual's responsibilities in a job description.[22]</li><li>Communicate this assigned role to the entire organization.</li></ul>	<ul><li>Is there a complete job description that accurately reflects assigned security duties and responsibilities?</li><li>Have the staff members in the organization been notified as to whom to call in the event of a security problem?[23]</li></ul>

---

[22] See Standard 4.22, *Standard: Documentation.*
[23] See Standard 4.5, *Security Awareness and Training*, and 4.6, *Security Incident Procedures.*

4.3. Workforce Security (§ 164.308(a)(3))

HIPAA Standard: *Implement policies and procedures to ensure that all members of its workforce have appropriate access to electronic protected health information, as provided under paragraph (a)(4) of this section, and to prevent those workforce members who do not have access under paragraph (a)(4) of this section from obtaining access to electronic protected health information.*

Key Activities	Description	Sample Questions
1. Implement Procedures for Authorization and/or Supervision Implementation Specification (Addressable)	• *Implement procedures for the authorization and/or supervision of workforce members who work with EPHI or in locations where it might be accessed.*	• Have chains of command and lines of authority been established? • Have staff members been made aware of the identity and roles of their supervisors?
2. Establish Clear Job Descriptions and Responsibilities[24]	• Define roles and responsibilities for all job functions. • Assign appropriate levels of security oversight, training, and access. • Identify in writing who has the business need—and who has been granted permission—to view, alter, retrieve, and store EPHI, and at what times, under what circumstances, and for what purposes.[25]	• Are there written job descriptions that are correlated with appropriate levels of access? • Have staff members been provided copies of their job descriptions, informed of the access granted to them, as well as the conditions by which this access can be used?
3. Establish Criteria and Procedures for Hiring and Assigning Tasks[26]	• Ensure that staff members have the necessary knowledge, skills, and abilities to fulfill particular roles, e.g., positions involving access to and use of sensitive information. • Ensure that these requirements are included as part of the personnel hiring process.	• Have the qualifications of candidates for specific positions been checked against the job description? • Have determinations been made that candidates for specific positions are able to perform the tasks of those positions?
4. Establish a Workforce Clearance Procedure Implementation Specification (Addressable)	• *Implement procedures to determine that the access of a workforce member to EPHI is appropriate.* • Implement appropriate screening of persons who will have access to EPHI. • Implement a procedure for obtaining clearance from appropriate offices or individuals where access is provided or terminated.	• Is there an implementation strategy that supports the designated access authorities? • Are applicants' employment and educational references checked, if reasonable and appropriate? • Have background checks been completed, if reasonable and appropriate? • Do procedures exist for obtaining appropriate sign-offs to grant or terminate access to EPHI?
5. Establish Termination Procedures Implementation Specification	• *Implement procedures for terminating access to EPHI when the employment of a workforce member ends or as required by determinations made as specified in*	• Are there separate procedures for voluntary termination (retirement, promotion, transfer, change of employment) vs. involuntary termination (termination for cause,

---

[24] See Key Activity 4.3.1, *Implement Procedures for Authorization and/or Supervision*. This activity and all associated bullets in the Description and Sample Questions are part of the procedures for authorization and/or supervision.
[25] See Section 4.22, *HIPAA Standard: Documentation*.
[26] See Key Activity 4.3.1, *Implement Procedures for Authorization and/or Supervision*. This activity and all associated bullets in the Description and Sample Questions are part of the procedures for authorization and/or supervision.

Key Activities	Description	Sample Questions
(Addressable)	§164.308(a)(3)(ii)(B). • Develop a standard set of procedures that should be followed to recover access control devices (Identification [ID] badges, keys, access cards, etc.) when employment ends. • Deactivate computer access accounts (e.g., disable user IDs and passwords). See the Access Controls Standard.	reduction in force, involuntary transfer, and criminal or disciplinary actions), if reasonable and appropriate? • Is there a standard checklist for all action items that should be completed when an employee leaves (return of all access devices, deactivation of logon accounts [including remote access], and delivery of any needed data solely under the employee's control)?

4.4. Information Access Management (§ 164.308(a)(4))[27]

HIPAA Standard: *Implement policies and procedures for authorizing access to electronic protected health information that are consistent with the applicable requirements of subpart E of this part.*

Key Activities	Description	Sample Questions
1. Isolate Healthcare Clearinghouse Functions[28] **Implementation Specification (Required)**	- If a healthcare clearinghouse is part of a larger organization, the clearinghouse must implement policies and procedures that protect the EPHI of the clearinghouse from unauthorized access by the larger organization. - Determine if a component of the covered entity constitutes a healthcare clearinghouse under the HIPAA Security Rule. - If no clearinghouse functions exist, document this finding. If a clearinghouse exists within the organization, implement procedures for access consistent with the HIPAA Privacy Rule.	- Does the healthcare clearinghouse share hardware or software with a larger organization of which it is a part? - Does the healthcare clearinghouse share staff or physical space with staff from a larger organization? - Has a separate network or subsystem been established for the healthcare clearinghouse, if reasonable and appropriate? - Has staff of the healthcare clearinghouse been trained to safeguard EPHI from disclosure to the larger organization, if required for compliance with the HIPAA Privacy Rule?
2. Implement Policies and Procedures for Authorizing Access **Implementation Specification (Addressable)**	- Implement policies and procedures for granting access to EPHI, for example, through access to a workstation, transaction, program, process, or other mechanism. - Decide how access will be granted to workforce members within the organization. - Select the basis for restricting access. - Select an access control method (e.g., identity-based, role-based, or other reasonable and appropriate means of access.) - Determine if direct access to EPHI will ever be appropriate for individuals external to the organization (e.g., business partners or patients seeking access to their own EPHI).	- Do the organization's IT systems have the capacity to set access controls?[29] - Are there documented job descriptions that accurately reflect assigned duties and responsibilities and enforce segregation of duties?[30] - Does the organization grant remote access to EPHI? - What method(s) of access control is (are) used (e.g., identity-based, role-based, location-based, or a combination)?
3. Implement Policies and Procedures for Access Establishment and Modification **Implementation Specification (Addressable)**	- Implement policies and procedures that, based upon the entity's access authorization policies, establish, document, review, and modify a user's right of access to a workstation, transaction, program, or process. - Establish standards for granting access. - Provide formal authorization from the appropriate authority before granting access to sensitive information.	- Are duties separated such that only the minimum necessary EPHI is made available to each staff member based on their job requirements?

---

[27] Note: See also Section 4.10, *HIPAA Standard: Facility Access Controls* and Section 4.14, *HIPAA Standard: Access Controls*.
[28] Note: Where the healthcare clearinghouse is a separate legal entity, it is subject to the Security Rule whether or not the larger organization is a covered entity.
[29] See Section 4.14, *HIPAA Standard: Access Controls*.
[30] See Section 4.3, *HIPAA Standard: Workforce Security*.

An Introductory Resource Guide for Implementing the Health Insurance Portability and Accountability Act (HIPAA) Security Rule

Key Activities	Description	Sample Questions
4. Evaluate Existing Security Measures Related to Access Controls[31]	• Evaluate the security features of access controls already in place, or those of any planned for implementation, as appropriate. • Determine if these security features involve alignment with other existing management, operational, and technical controls, such as policy standards and personnel procedures, maintenance and review of audit trails, identification and authentication of users, and physical access controls.	• Are there policies and procedures related to the security of access controls?[32] If so, are they updated regularly? • Are authentication mechanisms used to verify the identity of those accessing systems protected from inappropriate manipulation?[33] • Does management regularly review the list of access authorizations, including remote access authorizations, to verify that the list is accurate and has not been inappropriately altered?[34]

24

---

[31] See Key Activity 4.4.3, *Implement Policies and Procedures for Access Establishment and Modification*. This activity and all associated bullets in the Description and Sample Questions are part of the access establishment and modification implementation specification.
[32] See Section 4.22, *HIPAA Section: Documentation*.
[33] See Section 4.17, *HIPAA Standard: Person or Entity Authentication*.
[34] See Section 4.3, *HIPAA Standard: Workforce Security*.

4.5. Security Awareness and Training (§ 164.308(a)(5))[35]

HIPAA Standard: *Implement a security awareness and training program for all members of its workforce (including management).*

Key Activities	Description	Sample Questions
1. Conduct a Training Needs Assessment	• Determine the training needs of the organization. • Interview and involve key personnel in assessing security training needs.	• What awareness, training, and education programs are needed? Which are required? • What is the current status regarding how these needs are being addressed (e.g., how well are current efforts working)? • Where are the gaps between the needs and what is being done (e.g., what more needs to be done)? • What are the training priorities in terms of content and audience?
2. Develop and Approve a Training Strategy and a Plan	• Address the specific HIPAA policies that require security awareness and training in the security awareness and training program. • Outline in the security awareness and training program the scope of the awareness and training program; the goals; the target audiences; the learning objectives; the deployment methods, evaluation, and measurement techniques; and the frequency of training.	• Is there a procedure in place to ensure that everyone in the organization receives security awareness training? • What type of security training is needed to address specific technical topics based on job responsibility? • When should training be scheduled to ensure that compliance deadlines are met? • Has the organization considered the training needs of non-employees (e.g., contractors, interns)?

3. Protection from Malicious Software; Log-in Monitoring; and Password Management
 	
Implementation Specifications (All Addressable)
	• As reasonable and appropriate, train employees regarding procedures for:
	  ○ *Guarding against, detecting, and reporting malicious software;*
	  ○ *Monitoring log-in attempts and reporting discrepancies; and*
	  ○ *Creating changing, and safeguarding passwords.*
	• Incorporate information concerning staff members' roles and responsibilities in implementing these implementation specifications into training and awareness efforts.
		• Do employees know the importance of timely application of system patches to protect against malicious software and exploitation of vulnerabilities?
		• Are employees aware that log-in attempts may be monitored?
		• Do employees that monitor log-in attempts know to whom to report discrepancies?
		• Do employees understand their roles and responsibilities in selecting a password of appropriate strength, changing the password periodically (if required), and safeguarding their password?

4. Develop Appropriate Awareness and Training Content, Materials, and Methods	• Select topics that may need to be included in the training materials. • Incorporate new information from email advisories, online IT security daily news Web sites, and periodicals, as is reasonable and appropriate. • Consider using a variety of media and avenues according to what is appropriate for the organization based on workforce	• Have employees received a copy of, and do they have ready access to, the organization's security procedures and policies?[36] • Do employees know whom to contact and how to handle a security incident?[37] • Do employees understand the consequences of

---

[35] Note: See also Section 4.10, *HIPAA Standard: Facility Access Controls* and Section 4.14, *HIPAA Standard: Access Controls*.
[36] See Section 4.22, *HIPAA Standard: Documentation*.
[37] See Section 4.6, *HIPAA Standard: Security Incident Procedures*.

An Introductory Resource Guide for Implementing the Health Insurance Portability and Accountability Act (HIPAA) Security Rule

Key Activities	Description	Sample Questions
	size, location, level of education, etc.	• noncompliance with the stated security policies?[38] • Do employees who travel know how to handle physical laptop security issues and information security issues?[39] • Has the covered entity researched available training resources? • Is dedicated training staff available for delivery of security training? If not, who will deliver the training? • What is the security training budget?
5. Implement the Training	• Schedule and conduct the training outlined in the strategy and plan. • Implement any reasonable technique to disseminate the security messages in an organization, including newsletters, screensavers, videotapes, email messages, teleconferencing sessions, staff meetings, and computer-based training.	• Have all employees received adequate training to fulfill their security responsibilities? • Are there sanctions if employees do not complete required training?
6. Implement Security Reminders Implementation Specification (Addressable)	*Implement periodic security updates.* • Provide periodic security updates to staff, business associates, and contractors.	• What methods are available or already in use to make or keep employees aware of security, e.g., posters or booklets? • Is security refresher training performed on a periodic basis (e.g., annually)? • Is security awareness discussed with all new hires? • Are security topics reinforced during routine staff meetings?
7. Monitor and Evaluate Training Plan[40]	• Keep the security awareness and training program current. • Conduct training whenever changes occur in the technology and practices as appropriate. • Monitor the training program implementation to ensure that all employees participate. • Implement corrective actions when problems arise.[41]	• Are employee training and professional development programs documented and monitored, if reasonable and appropriate? • How are new employees trained on security? • Are new non-employees (e.g., contractors, interns) trained on security?

---

[38] See Section 4.1, *HIPAA Standard: Security Management Process.*
[39] See Section 4.13, *HIPAA Standard: Device and Media Controls.*
[40] Also required under the HIPAA Security Rule § 164.306, General Requirements, Subsection (e), *Maintenance.* See also Section 4.8, *HIPAA Standard: Evaluation.*
[41] See Section 4.1, *HIPAA Standard: Security Management Process.*

4.6. Security Incident Procedures (§ 164.308(a)(6))[42]

HIPAA Standard: *Implement policies and procedures to address security incidents.*

Key Activities	Description	Sample Questions
1. Determine Goals of Incident Response	• Gain an understanding as to what constitutes a true security incident. Under the HIPAA Security Rule, a security incident is the attempted or successful unauthorized access, use, disclosure, modification, or destruction of information or interference with system operations in an information system. (45 CFR § 164.304) • Determine how the organization will respond to a security incident. • Establish a reporting mechanism and a process to coordinate responses to the security incident. • Provide direct technical assistance, advise vendors to address product-related problems, and provide liaisons to legal and criminal investigative groups as needed.	• Has the HIPAA-required security risk assessment resulted in a list of potential physical or technological events that could result in a breach of security? • Is there a procedure in place for reporting and handling incidents? • Has an analysis been conducted that relates reasonably anticipated threats and hazards to the organization that could result in a security incident to the methods that would be used for mitigation? • Have the key functions of the organization been prioritized to determine what would need to be restored first in the event of a disruption?[43]
2. Develop and Deploy an Incident Response Team or Other Reasonable and Appropriate Response Mechanism	• Determine if the size, scope, mission, and other aspects of the organization justify the reasonableness and appropriateness of maintaining a standing incident response team. • Identify appropriate individuals to be a part of a formal incident response team, if the organization has determined that implementing an incident response team is reasonable and appropriate.	• Do members of the team have adequate knowledge of the organization's hardware and software? • Do members of the team have the authority to speak for the organization to the media, law enforcement, and clients or business partners? • Has the incident response team received appropriate training in incident response activities?
3. Develop and Implement Procedures to Respond to and Report Security Incidents **Implementation Specification (Required)**	• *Identify and respond to suspected or known security incidents; mitigate, to the extent practicable, harmful effects of security incidents that are known to the covered entity; and document security incidents and their outcomes.* • Document incident response procedures that can provide a single point of reference to guide the day-to-day operations of the incident response team. • Review incident response procedures with staff with roles and responsibilities related to incident response, solicit suggestions for improvements, and make changes to reflect input if reasonable and appropriate. • Update the procedures as required based on changing	• Has the organization determined that maintaining a staffed security incident hotline would be reasonable and appropriate? • Has the organization determined reasonable and appropriate mitigation options for security incidents? • Has the organization determined that standard incident report templates to ensure that all necessary information related to the incident is documented and investigated are reasonable and appropriate? • Has the organization determined under what conditions information related to a security breach will be disclosed to the media? • Have appropriate (internal and external) persons who

---

[42] Note: See also Section 4.10, *HIPAA Standard: Facility Access Controls* and Section 4.14, *HIPAA Standard: Access Controls.*
[43] See Section 4.7, *HIPAA Standard: Contingency Plan.*

An Introductory Resource Guide for Implementing the Health Insurance Portability and Accountability Act (HIPAA) Security Rule

Key Activities	Description	Sample Questions
	organizational needs.[44]	should be informed of a security breach been identified and a contact information list prepared? • Has a written incident response plan been developed and provided to the incident response team?
4. Incorporate Post-Incident Analysis into Updates and Revisions	• Measure effectiveness and update security incident response procedures to reflect lessons learned, and identify actions to take that will improve security controls after a security incident.	• Does the incident response team keep adequate documentation of security incidents and their outcomes, which may include what weaknesses were exploited and how access to information was gained? • Do records reflect new contacts and resources identified for responding to an incident? • Does the organization consider whether current procedures were adequate for responding to a particular security incident?

---

[44] See Section 4.22, *HIPAA Standard: Documentation.*

4.7. Contingency Plan (§ 164.308(a)(7)) [45]

HIPAA Standard: *Establish (and implement as needed) policies and procedures for responding to an emergency or other occurrence (for example, fire, vandalism, system failure, and natural disaster) that damages systems that contain electronic protected health information.*

Key Activities	Description	Sample Questions

1. **Develop Contingency Planning Policy**	• Define the organization's overall contingency objectives.
	• Establish the organizational framework, roles, and responsibilities for this area.
	• Address scope, resource requirements, training, testing, plan maintenance, and backup requirements.
	• A contingency planning methodology, based on NIST SP 800-34, is included in Appendix F of this document.
		• What critical services must be provided within specified timeframes?
		    ○ Patient treatment, for example, may need to be performed without disruption.
		    ○ By contrast, claims processing may be delayed during an emergency with no long-term damage to the organization.
		• Have cross-functional dependencies been identified so as to determine how the failure in one system may negatively impact another one?

2. **Conduct an Applications and Data Criticality Analysis** [46] **Implementation Specification (Addressable)**	• Assess the relative criticality of specific applications and data in support of other Contingency Plan components. • Identify the activities and material involving EPHI that are critical to business operations. • Identify the critical services or operations, and the manual and automated processes that support them, involving EPHI. • Determine the amount of time the organization can tolerate disruptions to these operations, material, or services (e.g., due to power outages). • Establish cost-effective strategies for recovering these critical services or processes.	• What hardware, software, and personnel are critical to daily operations? • What is the impact on desired service levels if these critical assets are not available? • What, if any, support is provided by external providers (Internet service providers [ISPs], utilities, or contractors)? • What is the nature and degree of impact on the operation if any of the critical resources are not available?
3. **Identify Preventive Measures** [47]	• Identify preventive measures for each defined scenario that could result in loss of a critical service operation involving the use of EPHI. • Ensure that identified preventive measures are practical and feasible in terms of their applicability in a given environment.	• What alternatives for continuing operations of the organization are available in case of loss of any critical function/resource? • What is the cost associated with the preventive measures that may be considered? • Are the preventive measures feasible (affordable and practical for the environment)? • What plans, procedures, or agreements need to be initiated to enable implementation of the preventive measures, if they are necessary?

---

[45] Note: See also Section 4.10, *HIPAA Standard: Facility Access Controls* and Section 4.14, *HIPAA Standard: Access Controls*.
[46] This activity may be conducted as part of a larger analysis, sometimes called an impact analysis, that considers all material, services, systems, processes, and activities, including those that do not involve EPHI and other elements of an organization not covered by the HIPAA Security Rule.
[47] See Key Activities 4.7.5, *Data Backup Plan and Disaster Recovery Plan* and 4.7.6, *Develop and Implement an Emergency Mode Operation Plan*. This activity and all associated bullets in the Description and Sample Questions are part of the data backup plan, disaster recovery plan and the emergency mode operation plan implementation specifications.

An Introductory Resource Guide for Implementing the Health Insurance Portability and Accountability Act (HIPAA) Security Rule

Key Activities	Description	Sample Questions
4. Develop Recovery Strategy[48]	• Finalize the set of contingency procedures that should be invoked for all identified impacts, including emergency mode operation. The strategy must be adaptable to the existing operating environment and address allowable outage times and associated priorities identified in step 2. • Ensure, if part of the strategy depends on external organizations for support, that formal agreements are in place with specific requirements stated.	• Have procedures related to recovery from emergency or disastrous events been documented? • Has a coordinator who manages, maintains, and updates the plan been designated? • Has an emergency call list been distributed to all employees? Have recovery procedures been documented? • Has a determination been made regarding when the plan needs to be activated (anticipated duration of outage, tolerances for outage or loss of capability, impact on service delivery, etc.)?
5. Data Backup Plan and Disaster Recovery Plan Implementation Specifications (Both Required)	• *Establish and implement procedures to create and maintain retrievable exact copies of EPHI.* • *Establish (and implement as needed) procedures to restore any loss of data.*	• Is there a formal, written contingency plan?[49] • Does it address disaster recovery and data backup?[50] • Do data backup procedures exist? • Are responsibilities assigned to conduct backup activities? • Are data backup procedures documented and available to other staff?
6. Develop and Implement an Emergency Mode Operation Plan Implementation Specification (Required)	• *Establish (and implement as needed) procedures to enable continuation of critical business processes for protection of the security of EPHI while operating in emergency mode. "Emergency mode" operation involves only those critical business processes that must occur to protect the security of EPHI during and immediately after a crisis situation.*	• Have procedures been developed to continue the critical functions identified in Key Activity? • If so, have those critical functions that also involve the use of EPHI been identified? • Would different staff, facilities, or systems be needed to perform those functions? • Has the security of that EPHI in that alternative mode of operation been assured?
7. Testing and Revision Procedure Implementation Specification (Addressable)	• *Implement procedures for periodic testing and revision of contingency plans.* • Test the contingency plan on a predefined cycle (stated in the policy developed under Key Activity), if reasonable and appropriate. • Train those with defined plan responsibilities on their roles. • If possible, involve external entities (vendors, alternative site/service providers) in testing exercises. • Make key decisions regarding how the testing is to occur ("tabletop" exercise versus staging a real operational scenario including actual loss of capability). • Decide how to segment the type of testing based on the assessment of business impact and acceptability of sustained loss of service. Consider cost.	• How is the plan to be tested? • Does testing lend itself to a phased approach? • Is it feasible to actually take down functions/services for the purposes of testing? • Can testing be done during normal business hours or must it take place during off hours? • If full testing is infeasible, has a "tabletop" scenario (e.g., a classroom-like exercise) been considered? • How frequently is the plan to be tested (e.g., annually)? • When should the plan be revised?

---

[48] See Key Activities 4.7.5, *Data Backup Plan and Disaster Recovery Plan* and 4.7.6, *Develop and Implement an Emergency Mode Operation Plan*. This activity and all associated bullets in the Description and Sample Questions are part of the data backup plan, disaster recovery plan and the emergency mode operation plan implementation specifications.
[49] See Key Activity 4.7.1, *Develop Contingency Planning Policy*.
[50] See Key Activity 4.7.1, *Develop Contingency Planning Policy*.

4.8. Evaluation (§ 164.308(a)(8))[51]

HIPAA Standard: *Perform a periodic technical and nontechnical evaluation, based initially upon the standards implemented under this rule and subsequently, in response to environmental or operational changes affecting the security of electronic protected health information, which establishes the extent to which an entity's security policies and procedures meet the requirements of this subpart.*

Key Activities	Description	Sample Questions
1. **Determine Whether Internal or External Evaluation Is Most Appropriate**	<ul><li>Decide whether the evaluation will be conducted with internal staff resources or external consultants.</li><li>Engage external expertise to assist the internal evaluation team where additional skills and expertise is determined to be reasonable and appropriate.</li><li>Use internal resources to supplement an external source of help, because these internal resources can provide the best institutional knowledge and history of internal policies and practices.</li></ul>	<ul><li>Which staff has the technical experience and expertise to evaluate the systems?</li><li>How much training will staff need on security-related technical and nontechnical issues?</li><li>If an outside vendor is used, what factors should be considered when selecting the vendor, such as credentials and experience?</li><li>What is the budget for internal resources to assist with an evaluation?</li><li>What is the budget for external services to assist with an evaluation?</li></ul>
2. **Develop Standards and Measurements for Reviewing All Standards and Implementation Specifications of the Security Rule**[52]	<ul><li>Use an evaluation strategy and tool that considers all elements of the HIPAA Security Rule and can be tracked, such as a questionnaire or checklist.</li><li>Implement tools that can provide reports on the level of compliance, integration, or maturity of a particular security safeguard deployed to protect EPHI.</li><li>If available, consider engaging corporate, legal, or regulatory compliance staff when conducting the analysis.</li><li>Leverage any existing reports or documentation that may already be prepared by the organization addressing compliance, integration, or maturity of a particular security safeguard deployed to protect EPHI.</li></ul>	<ul><li>Have management, operational, and technical issues been considered?</li><li>Do the elements of each evaluation procedure (questions, statements, or other components) address individual, measurable security safeguards for EPHI?</li><li>Has the organization determined that the procedure must be tested in a few areas or systems?</li><li>Does the evaluation tool consider all standards and implementation specifications of the HIPAA Security Rule?</li></ul>
3. **Conduct Evaluation**	<ul><li>Determine, in advance, what departments and/or staff will participate in the evaluation.</li><li>Secure management support for the evaluation process to ensure participation.</li><li>Collect and document all needed information. Collection methods may include the use of interviews, surveys, and outputs of automated tools, such as access control auditing tools, system logs, and results of penetration testing.</li><li>Conduct penetration testing (where trusted insiders attempt</li></ul>	<ul><li>If available, have staff members with knowledge of IT security been consulted and included in the evaluation team?</li><li>If penetration testing has been determined to be reasonable and appropriate, has specifically worded, written approval from senior management been received for any planned penetration testing?</li><li>Has the process been formally communicated to those who have been assigned roles and responsibilities in the</li></ul>

---

[51] Note: See also Section 4.10, *HIPAA Standard: Facility Access Controls* and Section 4.14, *HIPAA Standard: Access Controls*.
[52] Organizations may wish to review and employ, where reasonable and appropriate, security control assessment procedures found in NIST SP 800-53A, *Guide for Assessing the Security Controls in Federal Information Systems.*

An Introductory Resource Guide for Implementing the Health Insurance Portability and Accountability Act (HIPAA) Security Rule

Key Activities	Description	Sample Questions
	to compromise system security for the sole purpose of testing the effectiveness of security controls), if reasonable and appropriate.	evaluation process? • Has the organization explored the use of automated tools to support the evaluation process? • Has the organization employed automated tools to support the evaluation process?
4. Document Results[53]	• Document each evaluation finding, remediation options and recommendations, and remediation decisions. • Document known gaps between identified risks and mitigating security controls, and any acceptance of risk, including justification. • Develop security program priorities and establish targets for continuous improvement.	• Does the process support development of security recommendations? • In determining how best to display evaluation results, have written reports that highlight key findings and recommendations been considered? • If a written final report is to be circulated among key staff, have steps been taken to ensure that it is made available only to those persons designated to receive it?
5. Repeat Evaluations Periodically	• Establish the frequency of evaluations, taking into account the sensitivity of the EPHI controlled by the organization, its size, complexity, and environmental and/or operational changes (e.g., other relevant laws or accreditation requirements). • In addition to periodic reevaluations, consider repeating evaluations when environmental and operational changes are made to the organization that affects the security of EPHI (e.g., if new technology is adopted or if there are newly recognized risks to the security of the information).	• Do security policies specify that evaluations will be repeated when environmental and operational changes are made that affect the security of EPHI? • Do policies on frequency of security evaluations reflect any and all relevant federal or state laws which bear on environmental or operational changes affecting the security of EPHI? • Has the organization explored the use of automated tools to support periodic evaluations? • Has the organization employed automated tools to support periodic evaluations?

---

[53] See Section 4.22, *HIPAA Standard: Documentation.*

4.9. Business Associate Contracts and Other Arrangements (§ 164.308(b)(1))[54]

HIPAA Standard: *A covered entity, in accordance with § 164.306, may permit a business associate to create, receive, maintain, or transmit electronic protected health information on the covered entity's behalf only if the covered entity obtains satisfactory assurances, in accordance with § 164.314(a), that the business associate will appropriately safeguard the information*.[55,56]

Key Activities	Description	Sample Questions
1. Identify Entities that Are Business Associates under the HIPAA Security Rule	<ul><li>Identify the individual or department who will be responsible for coordinating the execution of business associate agreements or other arrangements.</li><li>Reevaluate the list of business associates to determine who has access to EPHI in order to assess whether the list is complete and current.</li><li>Identify systems covered by the contract/agreement.</li></ul>	<ul><li>Do the business associate agreements written and executed contain sufficient language to ensure that required information types will be protected?</li><li>Are there any new organizations or vendors that now provide a service or function on behalf of the organization? Such services may include the following:<ul><li>Claims processing or billing</li><li>Data analysis</li><li>Utilization review</li><li>Quality assurance</li><li>Benefit management</li><li>Practice management</li><li>Re-pricing</li><li>Hardware maintenance</li><li>All other HIPAA-regulated functions</li></ul></li><li>Have outsourced functions involving the use of EPHI been considered, such as the following:<ul><li>Actuarial services</li><li>Data aggregation</li><li>Administrative services</li><li>Accreditation</li><li>Financial services?</li></ul></li></ul>
2. Written Contract or Other Arrangement[57] Implementation Specification (Required)	<ul><li>Document the satisfactory assurances required by this standard through a written contract or other arrangement with the business associate that meets the applicable requirements of §164.314(a).[58]</li><li>Execute new or update existing agreements or arrangements as appropriate.</li><li>Identify roles and responsibilities.</li></ul>	<ul><li>Who is responsible for coordinating and preparing the final agreement or arrangement?</li><li>Does the agreement or arrangement specify how information is to be transmitted to and from the business associate?</li><li>Have security controls been specified for the business associate?</li></ul>

---

[54] See Section 4.19, *HIPAA Standard: Business Associate Contracts and Other Arrangements.*
[55] (2) This standard does not apply with respect to (i) the transmission by a covered entity of EPHI to a healthcare provider concerning the treatment of an individual; (ii) the transmission of EPHI by a group health plan or an HMO or health insurance issuer on behalf of a group health plan to a plan sponsor, to the extent that the requirements of §164.314(b) and §164.504(f) apply and are met; or (iii) the transmission of EPHI from or to other agencies providing the services at §164.502(e)(1)(ii)(C), when the covered entity is a health plan that is a government program providing public benefits, if the requirements of §164.502(e)(1)(ii)(C) are met.
[56] (3) A covered entity that violates the satisfactory assurances it provided as a business associate of another covered entity will be in noncompliance with the standards, implementation specifications, and requirements of this paragraph and §164.314(a).

Key Activities	Description	Sample Questions
	• Include security requirements in business associate contracts/agreements to address confidentiality, integrity, and availability of EPHI. • Specify any training requirements associated with the contract/agreement or arrangement, if reasonable and appropriate.	
3. Establish Process for Measuring Contract Performance and Terminating the Contract if Security Requirements Are Not Being Met[59]	• Maintain clear lines of communication. • Conduct periodic security reviews. • Establish criteria for measuring contract performance. • If the business associate is a governmental entity, update the memorandum of understanding or other arrangement when required by law or regulation or when reasonable and appropriate.	• What is the service being performed? • What is the outcome expected? • Is there a process for reporting security incidents related to the agreement? • Is there a process in place to periodically evaluate the effectiveness of business associate security controls? • Is there a process in place for terminating the contract if requirements are not being met and has the business associate been advised what conditions would warrant termination?
4. Implement An Arrangement Other than a Business Associate Contract if Reasonable and Appropriate	• If the covered entity and its business associate are both governmental entities, use a memorandum of understanding or reliance on law or regulation that requires equivalent actions on the part of the business associate. • Document the law, regulation, memorandum, or other document that assures that the governmental entity business associate will implement all required safeguards for EPHI involved in transactions between the parties.	• Is the covered entity's business associate a federal, state, or local governmental entity? • Is there a usual procedure for creating memoranda of understanding between the parties? • Has the covered entity researched and reviewed all law and regulation governing the use of EPHI by the governmental entity business associate?

---

[57] See also Key Activity 4.9.4, *Implement an Arrangement Other than a Business Associate Contract if Reasonable and Appropriate.*
[58] See Section 4.19, *HIPAA Standard: Business Associate Contracts and Other Arrangements.*
[59] See Section 4.19, *HIPAA Standard: Business Associate Contracts and Other Arrangements.*

An Introductory Resource Guide for Implementing the HIPAA Security Rule

Physical Safeguards

4.10. Facility Access Controls (§ 164.310(a)(1))[60]

HIPAA Standard: *Implement policies and procedures to limit physical access to its electronic information systems and the facility or facilities in which they are housed, while ensuring that properly authorized access is allowed.*

	Key Activities	Description	Sample Questions
1.	Conduct an Analysis of Existing Physical Security Vulnerabilities[61, 62]	<ul><li>Inventory facilities and identify shortfalls and/or vulnerabilities in current physical security capabilities.</li><li>Assign degrees of significance to each vulnerability identified and ensure that proper access is allowed.</li><li>Determine which types of facilities require access controls to safeguard EPHI, such as:<ul><li>Data Centers</li><li>Peripheral equipment locations</li><li>IT staff offices</li><li>Workstation locations.</li></ul></li></ul>	<ul><li>If reasonable and appropriate, do nonpublic areas have locks and cameras?</li><li>Are workstations protected from public access or viewing?[63]</li><li>Are entrances and exits that lead to locations with EPHI secured?</li><li>Do policies and procedures already exist regarding access to and use of facilities and equipment?</li><li>Are there possible natural or man-made disasters that could happen in our environment?[64]</li><li>Do normal physical protections exist (locks on doors, windows, etc., and other means of preventing unauthorized access)?</li></ul>
2.	Identify Corrective Measures[65, 66]	<ul><li>Identify and assign responsibility for the measures and activities necessary to correct deficiencies and ensure that proper access is allowed.</li><li>Develop and deploy policies and procedures to ensure that repairs, upgrades, and /or modifications are made to the appropriate physical areas of the facility while ensuring that proper access is allowed.</li></ul>	<ul><li>Who is responsible for security?[67]</li><li>Is a workforce member other than the security official responsible for facility/physical security?</li><li>Are facility access control policies and procedures already in place? Do they need to be revised?</li><li>What training will be needed for employees to understand the policies and procedures?[68]</li><li>How will we document the decisions and actions?[69]</li><li>Are we dependent on a landlord to make physical changes to meet the requirements?</li></ul>

---

[60] Note: See also Section 4.10, *HIPAA Standard: Facility Access Controls* and Section 4.14, *HIPAA Standard: Access Controls*.
[61] This key activity may be performed as part of the risk analysis implementation specification. See Section 4.1, *HIPAA Standard: Security Management Process*.
[62] See Key Activity 4.10.3, *Develop a Facility Security Plan*. This activity and all associated bullets in the Description and Sample Questions are part of the facility security plan implementation specification.
[63] See Section 4.11, *HIPAA Standard: Workstation Use*.
[64] See Section 4.7, *HIPAA Standard: Contingency Plan*.
[65] This key activity may be performed as part of the risk management implementation specification. See Section 4.1, *HIPAA Standard: Security Management Process*.
[66] See Key Activity 4.10.3, *Develop a Facility Security Plan*. This activity and all associated bullets in the Description and Sample Questions are part of the facility security plan implementation specification.
[67] See Section 4.2, *HIPAA Standard: Assigned Security Responsibility*.
[68] See Section 4.5, *HIPAA Standard: Security Awareness and Training*.

An Introductory Resource Guide for Implementing the HIPAA Security Rule

Key Activities	Description	Sample Questions
3. Develop a Facility Security Plan Implementation Specification (Addressable)	• *Implement policies and procedures to safeguard the facility and the equipment therein from unauthorized physical access, tampering, and theft.* • Implement appropriate measures to provide physical security protection for EPHI in a covered entity's possession. • Include documentation of the facility inventory, as well as information regarding the physical maintenance records and the history of changes, upgrades, and other modifications. • Identify points of access to the facility and existing security controls.	• Is there an inventory of facilities and existing security practices? • What are the current procedures for securing the facilities (exterior, interior, equipment, access controls, maintenance records, etc.)? • Is a workforce member other than the security official responsible for the facility plan? • Is there a contingency plan already in place, under revision, or under development?[70]
4. Develop Access Control and Validation Procedures Implementation Specification (Addressable)	• *Implement procedures to control and validate a person's access to facilities based on their role or function, including visitor control, and control of access to software programs for testing and revision.* • Implement procedures to provide facility access to authorized personnel and visitors, and exclude unauthorized persons.	• What are the policies and procedures in place for controlling access by staff, contractors, visitors, and probationary employees? • How many access points exist in each facility? Is there an inventory? • Is monitoring equipment necessary?
5. Establish Contingency Operations Procedures Implementation Specification (Addressable)	• *Establish (and implement as needed) procedures that allow facility access in support of restoration of lost data under the Disaster Recovery Plan and Emergency Mode Operations Plan in the event of an emergency.*	• Who needs access to EPHI in the event of a disaster? • What is the backup plan for access to the facility and/or EPHI? • Who is responsible for the contingency plan for access to EPHI? • Who is responsible for implementing the contingency plan for access to EPHI in each department, unit, etc.? • Will the contingency plan be appropriate in the event of all types of potential disasters (fire, flood, earthquake, etc.)?
6. Maintain Maintenance Records Implementation Specification (Addressable)	• *Implement policies and procedures to document repairs and modifications to the physical components of a facility which are related to security (for example, hardware, walls, doors and locks).*	• Are records of repairs to hardware, walls, doors, and locks maintained? • Has responsibility for maintaining these records been assigned?

---

[69] See Section 4.22, *HIPAA Standard: Documentation.*
[70] See Section 4.7, *HIPAA Standard: Contingency Plan.*

An Introductory Resource Guide for Implementing the HIPAA Security Rule

4.11. Workstation Use (§ 164.310(b))

HIPAA Standard: *Implement policies and procedures that specify the proper functions to be performed, the manner in which those functions are to be performed, and the physical attributes of the surroundings of a specific workstation or class of workstation that can access electronic protected health information.*

Key Activities	Description	Sample Questions
1. Identify Workstation Types and Functions or Uses	<ul><li>Inventory workstations and devices.</li><li>Develop policies and procedures for each type of workstation and workstation device, identifying and accommodating their unique issues.</li><li>Classify workstations based on the capabilities, connections, and allowable activities for each workstation used.</li></ul>	<ul><li>Do we have an inventory of workstation types and locations in my organization?</li><li>Who is responsible for this inventory and its maintenance?</li><li>What tasks are commonly performed on a given workstation or type of workstation?</li><li>Are all types of computing devices used as workstations identified along with the use of these workstations?</li></ul>
2. Identify Expected Performance of Each Type of Workstation	<ul><li>Develop and document policies and procedures related to the proper use and performance of workstations.</li></ul>	<ul><li>How are workstations used in day-to-day operations?</li><li>What are key operational risks that could result in a breach of security?</li></ul>
3. Analyze Physical Surroundings for Physical Attributes[71]	<ul><li>Ensure that any risks associated with a workstation's surroundings are known and analyzed for possible negative impacts.</li><li>Develop policies and procedures that will prevent or preclude unauthorized access of unattended workstations, limit the ability of unauthorized persons to view sensitive information, and dispose of sensitive information as needed.</li></ul>	<ul><li>Where are workstations located?</li><li>Is viewing by unauthorized individuals restricted or limited at these workstations?</li><li>Do changes need to be made in the space configuration?</li><li>Do employees understand the security requirements for the data they use in their day-to-day jobs?</li></ul>

---

[71] See Section 4.5, *HIPAA Standard: Security Awareness and Training*. This key activity should be performed during security training or awareness activities.

4.12. Workstation Security (§ 164.310(c))

HIPAA Standard: *Implement physical safeguards for all workstations that access electronic protected health information, to restrict access to authorized users.*

Key Activities	Description	Sample Questions
1. Identify All Methods of Physical Access to Workstations	• Document the different ways workstations are accessed by employees and nonemployees.	• Is there an inventory of all current workstation locations? • Are any workstations located in public areas? • Are laptops used as workstations?
2. Analyze the Risk Associated with Each Type of Access[72]	• Determine which type of access holds the greatest threat to security.	• Are any workstations in areas that are more vulnerable to unauthorized use, theft, or viewing of the data they contain? • What are the options for making modifications to the current access configuration?
3. Identify and Implement Physical Safeguards for Workstations	• Implement physical safeguards and other security measures to minimize the possibility of inappropriate access to EPHI through workstations.	• What safeguards are in place, i.e., locked doors, screen barriers, cameras, guards?[73] • Do any workstations need to be relocated to enhance physical security? • Have employees been trained on security?[74]

---

[72] This key activity may be conducted pursuant to the risk analysis and risk management implementation specifications of the security management process standard. See Section 4.1, *HIPAA Standard: Security Management Process.*
[73] See Section 4.1, *HIPAA Standard: Security Management Process.*
[74] See Section 4.5, *HIPAA Standard: Security Awareness and Training.*

An Introductory Resource Guide for Implementing the HIPAA Security Rule

4.13. Device and Media Controls (§ 164.310(d)(1))

HIPAA Standard: *Implement policies and procedures that govern the receipt and removal of hardware and electronic media that contain electronic protected health information into and out of a facility, and the movement of these items within the facility.*

Key Activities	Description	Sample Questions
1. Implement Methods for Final Disposal of EPHI Implementation Specification (Required)	• *Implement policies and procedures to address the final disposition of EPHI and/or the hardware or electronic media on which it is stored.* • Determine and document the appropriate methods to dispose of hardware, software, and the data itself. • Assure that EPHI is properly destroyed and cannot be recreated.	• What data is maintained by the organization, and where? • Is data on removable, reusable media such as tapes and CDs? • Is there a process for destroying data on hard drives and file servers? • What are the options for disposing of data on hardware? What are the costs?
2. Develop and Implement Procedures for Reuse of Electronic Media Implementation Specification (Required)	• *Implement procedures for removal of EPHI from electronic media before the media are made available for reuse.* • Ensure that EPHI previously stored on electronic media cannot be accessed and reused. • Identify removable media and their use. • Ensure that EPHI is removed from reusable media before they are used to record new information.	• Do policies and procedures already exist regarding reuse of electronic media (hardware and software)? • Is one individual and/or department responsible for coordinating the disposal of data and the reuse of the hardware and software? • Are employees appropriately trained on security and risks to EPHI when reusing software and hardware?[75]
3. Maintain Accountability for Hardware and Electronic Media Implementation Specification (Addressable)	• *Maintain a record of the movements of hardware and electronic media and any person responsible therefore.* • Ensure that EPHI is not inadvertently released or shared with any unauthorized party. • Ensure that an individual is responsible for, and records the receipt and removal of, hardware and software with EPHI.	• Where is data stored (what type of media)? • What procedures already exist regarding tracking of hardware and software within the company? • If workforce members are allowed to remove electronic media that contain or may be used to access EPHI, do procedures exist to track the media externally? • Who is responsible for maintaining records of hardware and software?
4. Develop Data Backup and Storage Procedures Implementation Specification (Addressable)	• *Create a retrievable exact copy of EPHI, when needed, before movement of equipment.* • Ensure that an exact retrievable copy of the data is retained and protected to protect the integrity of EPHI during equipment relocation.	• Are backup files maintained offsite to assure data availability in the event data is lost while transporting or moving electronic media containing EPHI? • If data were to be unavailable while media are transported or moved for a period of time, what would the business impact be?

---

[75] See Section 4.5, *HIPAA Standard: Security Awareness and Training*.

An Introductory Resource Guide for Implementing the HIPAA Security Rule

Technical Safeguards

4.14. Access Control (§ 164.312(a)(1))

HIPAA Standard: *Implement technical policies and procedures for electronic information systems that maintain electronic protected health information to allow access only to those persons or software programs that have been granted access rights as specified in § 164.308(a)(4).*[76]

Key Activities	Description	Sample Questions
1. Analyze Workloads and Operations To Identify the Access Needs of All Users [77]	• Identify an approach for access control. • Consider all applications and systems containing EPHI that should be available only to authorized users. • Integrate these activities into the access granting and management process. [78]	• Have all applications/systems with EPHI been identified? • What user roles are defined for those applications/systems? • Where is the EPHI supporting those applications/systems currently housed (e.g., stand-alone PC, network)? • Are data and/or systems being accessed remotely?
2. Identify Technical Access Control Capabilities	• Determine the access control capability of all information systems with EPHI.	• How are the systems accessed (viewing data, modifying data, creating data)?
3. Ensure that All System Users Have Been Assigned a Unique Identifier *Implementation Specification (Required)*	• Assign a unique name and/or number for identifying and tracking user identity. • Ensure that system activity can be traced to a specific user. • Ensure that the necessary data is available in the system logs to support audit and other related business functions. [79]	• How should the identifier be established (length and content)? • Should the identifier be self-selected or randomly generated?
4. Develop Access Control Policy [80]	• Establish a formal policy for access control that will guide the development of procedures. [81] • Specify requirements for access control that are both feasible and cost-effective for implementation. [82]	• Have rules of behavior been established and communicated to system users? • How will rules of behavior be enforced?
5. Implement Access Control Procedures Using Selected Hardware and Software	• Implement the policy and procedures using existing or additional hardware/software solution(s).	• Who will manage the access controls procedures? • Are current users trained in access control management? [83] • Will user training be needed to implement access control procedures?

---

[76] Note: This HIPAA standard supports the standards at Section 4.4, *Information Access Management* and Section 4.10, *Facility Access Controls*.
[77] See Section 4.4, *HIPAA Standard: Information Access Management*. This activity and all associated bullets in the Description and Sample Questions should be conducted as part of the access granting and access establishment process detailed in the Information Access Management standard.
[78] See Section 4.4, *HIPAA Standard: Information Access Management*.
[79] See Section 4.15, *HIPAA Standard: Audit Control*.
[80] See Section 4.4, *HIPAA Standard: Information Access Management*.
[81] See Section 4.4, *HIPAA Standard: Information Access Management*.
[82] See Section 4.1, *HIPAA Standard: Security Management Process*.

An Introductory Resource Guide for Implementing the HIPAA Security Rule

	Key Activities	Description	Sample Questions
6.	**Review and Update User Access**	<ul><li>Enforce policy and procedures as a matter of ongoing operations.[84]</li><li>Determine if any changes are needed for access control mechanisms.</li><li>Establish procedures for updating access when users require the following:[85]<ul><li>○ Initial access</li><li>○ Increased access</li><li>○ Access to different systems or applications than those they currently have</li></ul></li></ul>	<ul><li>Have new employees/users been given proper instructions for protecting data and systems?[86]</li><li>What are the procedures for new employee/user access to data and systems?[87]</li><li>Are there procedures for reviewing and, if appropriate, modifying access authorizations for existing users?[88]</li></ul>
7.	**Establish an Emergency Access Procedure** **Implementation Specification (Required)**	<ul><li>*Establish (and implement as needed) procedures for obtaining necessary electronic protected health information during an emergency.*</li><li>Identify a method of supporting continuity of operations should the normal access procedures be disabled or unavailable due to system problems.</li></ul>	<ul><li>When should the emergency access procedure be activated?</li><li>Who is authorized to make the decision?[89]</li><li>Who has assigned roles in the process?[90]</li><li>Will systems automatically default to settings and functionalities that will enable the emergency access procedure or will the mode be activated by the system administrator or other authorized individual?</li></ul>
8.	**Automatic Logoff and Encryption and Decryption** **Implementation Specifications (Both Addressable)**	<ul><li>Consider whether the addressable implementation specifications of this standard are reasonable and appropriate:<ul><li>○ *Implement electronic procedures that terminate an electronic session after a predetermined time of inactivity.*</li><li>○ *Implement a mechanism to encrypt and decrypt EPHI.*</li></ul></li></ul>	<ul><li>Are automatic logoff features available for any of the covered entity's operating systems or other major applications?</li><li>If applications have been created or developed in-house, is it reasonable and appropriate to modify them to feature automatic logoff capability?</li><li>What period of inactivity prior to automatic logoff is reasonable and appropriate for the covered entity?</li><li>What encryption systems are available for the covered entity's EPHI?</li><li>Is encryption appropriate for storing and maintaining EPHI ("at rest"), as well as while it is transmitted?</li></ul>
9.	**Terminate Access if it is No Longer Required**[91]	<ul><li>Ensure that access to EPHI is terminated if the access is no longer authorized.</li></ul>	<ul><li>Are rules being enforced to remove access by staff members who no longer have a need to know because they have changed assignments or have stopped working for the organization?</li></ul>

---

[83] See Section 4.5, *HIPAA Standard: Security Awareness and Training.*
[84] See Section 4.4, *HIPAA Standard: Information Access Management.*
[85] See Section 4.4, *HIPAA Standard: Information Access Management.*
[86] See Section 4.5, *HIPAA Standard: Security Awareness and Training.*
[87] See Section 4.4, *HIPAA Standard: Information Access Management.*
[88] See Section 4.4, *HIPAA Standard: Information Access Management.*
[89] See Section 4.7, *HIPAA Standard: Contingency Plan.*
[90] See Section 4.7, *HIPAA Standard: Contingency Plan.*
[91] See Section 4.3, *HIPAA Standard: Workforce Security.*

An Introductory Resource Guide for Implementing the HIPAA Security Rule

4.15. Audit Controls (§ 164.312(b))

HIPAA Standard: *Implement hardware, software, and/or procedural mechanisms that record and examine activity in information systems that contain or use electronic protected health information.*

Key Activities	Description	Sample Questions
1. **Determine the Activities that Will Be Tracked or Audited**	• Determine the appropriate scope of audit controls that will be necessary in information systems that contain or use EPHI based on the covered entity's risk assessment and other organizational factors.[92] • Determine what data needs to be captured.	• Where is EPHI at risk in the organization?[93] • What systems, applications, or processes make data vulnerable to unauthorized or inappropriate tampering, uses, or disclosures?[94] • What activities will be monitored (e.g., creation, reading, updating, and/or deleting of files or records containing EPHI)? • What should the audit record include (e.g., user ID, event type/date/time)?
2. **Select the Tools that Will Be Deployed for Auditing and System Activity Reviews**	• Evaluate existing system capabilities and determine if any changes or upgrades are necessary.	• What tools are in place? • What are the most appropriate monitoring tools for the organization (third party, freeware, or operating system-provided)? • Are changes/upgrades to information systems reasonable and appropriate?
3. **Develop and Deploy the Information System Activity Review/Audit Policy**	• Document and communicate to the workforce the facts about the organization's decisions on audits and reviews.	• Who is responsible for the overall audit process and results? • How often will audits take place? • How often will audit results be analyzed? • What is the organization's sanction policy for employee violations?[95] • Where will audit information reside (i.e., separate server)?
4. **Develop Appropriate Standard Operating Procedures**[96]	• Determine the types of audit trail data and monitoring procedures that will be needed to derive exception reports.	• How will exception reports or logs be reviewed? • Where will monitoring reports be filed and maintained? • Is there a formal process in place to address system misuse, abuse, and fraudulent activity?[97] • How will managers and employees be notified, when appropriate, regarding suspect activity?

---

[92] See Section 4.1, *HIPAA Standard: Security Management Process* and Key Activity 4.1.7, *Develop and Deploy the Information System Activity Review Process*.
[93] See Section 4.1, *HIPAA Standard: Security Management Process* and Key Activity 4.1.2, *Conduct Risk Assessment*.
[94] See Section 4.1, *HIPAA Standard: Security Management Process* and Key Activity 4.1.2, *Conduct Risk Assessment*.
[95] See Section 4.1, *HIPAA Standard: Security Management Process* and Key Activity 4.1.6, *Develop and Implement a Sanction Policy*.
[96] See Section 4.1, *HIPAA Standard: Security Management Process* and Key Activity 4.1.7, *Develop and Deploy the Information system Activity Review Process*..
[97] See Section 4.1, *HIPAA Standard: Security Management Process* and Key Activity 4.1.6, *Develop and Implement a Sanction Policy*.

An Introductory Resource Guide for Implementing the HIPAA Security Rule

Key Activities	Description	Sample Questions
5. Implement the Audit/System Activity Review Process[98]	<ul><li>Activate the necessary audit system.</li><li>Begin logging and auditing procedures.</li></ul>	<ul><li>What mechanisms will be implemented to assess the effectiveness of the audit process (metrics)?</li><li>What is the plan to revise the audit process when needed?</li></ul>

---

[98] See Section 4.1, *HIPAA Standard: Security Management Process* and Key Activity 4.1.9, *Implement the Information System Activity Review and Audit Process*.

An Introductory Resource Guide for Implementing the HIPAA Security Rule

4.16. Integrity (§ 164.312(c)(1))

HIPAA Standard: *Implement policies and procedures to protect electronic protected health information from improper alteration or destruction.*

	Key Activities	Description	Sample Questions
1.	Identify All Users Who Have Been Authorized to Access EPHI[99]	• Identify all approved users with the ability to alter or destroy data, if reasonable and appropriate. • Address this Key Activity in conjunction with the identification of unauthorized sources in Key Activity 2, below.	• How are users authorized to access the information?[100] • Is there a sound basis established as to why they need the access?[101] • Have they been trained on how to use the information?[102] • Is there an audit trail established for all accesses to the information?[103]
2.	Identify Any Possible Unauthorized Sources that May Be Able to Intercept the Information and Modify It	• Identify scenarios that may result in modification to the EPHI by unauthorized sources (e.g., hackers, disgruntled employees, business competitors).[104] • Conduct this activity as part of your risk analysis.[105]	• What are likely sources that could jeopardize information integrity?[106] • What can be done to protect the integrity of the information when it is residing in a system (at rest)? • What procedures and policies can be established to decrease or eliminate alteration of the information during transmission (e.g., encryption)?[107]
3.	Develop the Integrity Policy and Requirements	• Establish a formal (written) set of integrity requirements based on the results of the analysis completed in the previous steps.	• Have the requirements been discussed and agreed to by identified key personnel involved in the processes that are affected? • Have the requirements been documented? • Has a written policy been developed and communicated to system users?
4.	Implement Procedures to Address These Requirements	• Identify and implement methods that will be used to protect the information from modification. • Identify and implement tools and techniques to be developed or procured that support the assurance of integrity.	• Are current audit, logging, and access control techniques sufficient to address the integrity of the information? • If not, what additional techniques can we apply to check information integrity (e.g., quality control process, transaction and output reconstruction)?

---

[99] See Section 4.3, HIPAA Standard: *Workforce Security*, Section 4.3, HIPAA Standard: *Access Control*, and Section 4.21, HIPAA Standard: *Policies and Procedures.*
[100] See Section 4.3, HIPAA Standard: *Workforce Security* and Section 4.3, HIPAA Standard: *Access Control.*
[101] See Section 4.3, HIPAA Standard: *Workforce Security.*
[102] See Section 4.5, HIPAA Standard: *Security Awareness and Training.*
[103] See Section 4.15, HIPAA Standard: *Audit Controls.*
[104] See Section 4.1, HIPAA Standard: *Security Management Process.*
[105] See Section 4.1, HIPAA Standard: *Security Management Process.*
[106] See Section 4.1, HIPAA Standard: *Security Management Process.*
[107] See Section 4.1, HIPAA Standard: *Security Management Process.*

An Introductory Resource Guide for Implementing the HIPAA Security Rule

Key Activities	Description	Sample Questions
		• Can additional training of users decrease instances attributable to human errors?
5. Implement a Mechanism to Authenticate EPHI Implementation Specification (Addressable)	• *Implement electronic mechanisms to corroborate that EPHI has not been altered or destroyed in an unauthorized manner.* • Consider possible electronic mechanisms for authentication such as: 　○ Error-correcting memory 　○ Magnetic disk storage 　○ Digital signatures 　○ Check sum technology.	• Are the uses of both electronic and nonelectronic mechanisms necessary for the protection of EPHI? • Are appropriate electronic authentication tools available? • Are available electronic authentication tools interoperable with other applications and system components?
6. Establish a Monitoring Process To Assess How the Implemented Process Is Working	• Review existing processes to determine if objectives are being addressed.[108] • Reassess integrity processes continually as technology and operational environments change to determine if they need to be revised.[109]	• Are there reported instances of information integrity problems and have they decreased since integrity procedures have been implemented?[110] • Does the process, as implemented, provide a higher level of assurance that information integrity is being maintained?

---

[108] See Section 4.8, *HIPAA Standard: Evaluation.*
[109] See Section 4.8, *HIPAA Standard: Evaluation.*
[110] See Section 4.6, *HIPAA Standard: Security Incident Procedures.*

4.17. Person or Entity Authentication (§ 164.312(d))[111]

HIPAA Standard: *Implement procedures to verify that a person or entity seeking access to electronic protected health information is the one claimed.*

Key Activities	Description	Sample Questions
1. **Determine Authentication Applicability to Current Systems/Applications**	• Identify methods available for authentication. Under the HIPAA Security Rule, authentication is the corroboration that a person is the one claimed. (45 CFR § 164.304). • Authentication requires establishing the validity of a transmission source and/or verifying an individual's claim that he or she has been authorized for specific access privileges to information and information systems.	• What authentication methods are available? • What are the advantages and disadvantages of each method? • What will it cost to implement the available methods in our environment? • Do we have trained staff who can maintain the system or do we need to consider outsourcing some of the support? • Are passwords being used? • If so, are they unique by individual?
2. **Evaluate Authentication Options Available**	• Weigh the relative advantages and disadvantages of commonly used authentication approaches. • There are four commonly used authentication approaches available: 　○ Something a person knows, such as a password, 　○ Something a person has or is in possession of, such as a token (smart card, ATM card, etc.), 　○ Some type of biometric identification a person provides, such as a fingerprint, or 　○ A combination of two or more of the above approaches.	• What are the strengths and weaknesses of each available option? • Which can be best supported with assigned resources (budget/staffing)? • What level of authentication is appropriate based on our assessment of risk to the information/systems? • Do we need to acquire outside vendor support to implement the process?
3. **Select and Implement Authentication Option**	• Consider the results of the analysis conducted under Key Activity 2, above, and select appropriate authentication methods. • Implement the methods selected into your operations and activities.	• Has necessary user and support staff training been completed? • Have formal authentication policy and procedures been established and communicated? • Has necessary testing been completed to ensure that the authentication system is working as prescribed? • Do the procedures include ongoing system maintenance and updates? • Is the process implemented in such a way that it does not compromise the authentication information (password file encryption, etc.)?

---

[111] See also Section 4.14, *HIPAA Standard: Access Control* and Section 4.15, *HIPAA Standard: Audit Controls.*

An Introductory Resource Guide for Implementing the HIPAA Security Rule

4.18. Transmission Security (§ 164.312(e)(1))

HIPAA Standard: *Implement technical security measures to guard against unauthorized access to electronic protected health information that is being transmitted over an electronic communications network.*

Key Activities	Description	Sample Questions
1. Identify Any Possible Unauthorized Sources that May Be Able to Intercept and/or Modify the Information	• Identify scenarios that may result in modification of the EPHI by unauthorized sources during transmission (e.g., hackers, disgruntled employees, business competitors).[112]	• What measures exist to protect EPHI in transmission? • Is there an auditing process in place to verify that EPHI has been protected against unauthorized access during transmission?[113] • Are there trained staff members to monitor transmissions?
2. Develop and Implement Transmission Security Policy and Procedures	• Establish a formal (written) set of requirements for transmitting EPHI. • Identify methods of transmission that will be used to safeguard EPHI. • Identify tools and techniques that will be used to support the transmission security policy. • Implement procedures for transmitting EPHI using hardware and/or software, if needed.	• Have the requirements been discussed and agreed to by identified key personnel involved in transmitting EPHI? • Has a written policy been developed and communicated to system users?
3. Implement Integrity Controls *Implementation Specification (Addressable)*	*Implement security measures to ensure that electronically transmitted EPHI is not improperly modified without detection until disposed of.*	• What measures are planned to protect EPHI in transmission? • Is there assurance that information is not altered during transmission?
4. Implement Encryption *Implementation Specification (Addressable)*	*Implement a mechanism to encrypt EPHI whenever deemed appropriate.*	• Is encryption reasonable and appropriate for EPHI in transmission? • Is encryption needed to effectively protect the information in transmission? • Is encryption feasible and cost-effective in this environment? • What encryption algorithms and mechanisms are available? • Does the covered entity have the appropriate staff to maintain a process for encrypting EPHI during transmission? • Are staff members skilled in the use of encryption?

---

[112] See Section 4.7, *HIPAA Standard: Contingency Plan* and Section 4.1, *HIPAA Standard: Security Management Process.*
[113] See Section 4.1, *HIPAA Standard: Security Management Process.*

Organizational Requirements

4.19. Business Associate Contracts or Other Arrangements (§ 164.314(a)(1))

HIPAA Standard: *(i) The contract or other arrangement between the covered entity and its business associate required by § 164.308(b) must meet the requirements of paragraph (a)(2)(i) or (a)(2)(ii) of this section, as applicable. (ii) A covered entity is not in compliance with the standards in § 164.502(e) and paragraph (a) of this section if the covered entity knew of a pattern of an activity or practice of the business associate that constituted a material breach or violation of the business associate's obligation under the contract or other arrangement, unless the covered entity took reasonable steps to cure the breach or end the violation, as applicable, and, if such steps were unsuccessful—(A) Terminated the contract or arrangement, if feasible; or (B) If termination is not feasible, reported the problem to the Secretary.*

Key Activities	Description	Sample Questions
1. Contract Must Provide that Business Associates Adequately Protect EPHI[114] **Implementation Specification (Required)**	• *Contracts between covered entities and business associates must provide that business associates will implement administrative, physical, and technical safeguards that reasonably and appropriately protect the confidentiality, integrity, and availability of the EPHI that the business associate creates, receives, maintains, or transmits on behalf of the covered entity.* • *May consider asking the business associate to conduct a risk assessment that addresses administrative, technical, and physical risks, if reasonable and appropriate.*	• Does the written agreement between the covered entity and the business associate address the applicable functions related to creating, receiving, maintaining, and transmitting EPHI that the business associate is to perform on behalf of the covered entity?
2. Contract Must Provide that Business Associate's Agents Adequately Protect EPHI **Implementation Specification (Required)**	• *Contracts between covered entities and business associates must provide that any agent, including a subcontractor, to whom the business associate provides such information agrees to implement reasonable and appropriate safeguards to protect it;*	• Does the written agreement address the issue of EPHI access by subcontractors and other agents of the business associate?
3. Contract Must Provide that Business Associates will Report Security Incidents **Implementation Specification (Required)**	• *Contracts between covered entities and business associates must provide that business associates will report to the covered entity any security incident of which it becomes aware.* • *Establish a reporting mechanism and a process for the business associate to use in the event of a security incident.*	• Is there a procedure in place for reporting of incidents by business associates? • Have key business associate staff that would be the point of contact in the event of a security incident been identified?

---

[114] Note that business associate contracts must also comply with provisions of the HIPAA Privacy Rule. See 45 CFR, Part 164 — *Security and Privacy* § 164.504(e) *(Standard: Business associate contracts).*

An Introductory Resource Guide for Implementing the HIPAA Security Rule

Key Activities	Description	Sample Questions

4. Contract Must Provide that Business Associate Will Authorize Termination of the Contract if it has been Materially Breached
 	
Implementation Specification (Required)
	• *Contracts between covered entities and business associates must provide that the business associate will authorize termination of the contract by the covered entity if the covered entity determines that the business associate has violated a material term of the contract.*
	• Establish in the written agreement with business associates the circumstances under which a violation of agreements relating to the security of EPHI constitutes a material breach of the contract.
	• Terminate the contract if:
	   ○ the covered entity learns that the business associate has violated the contract or materially breached it, and
	   ○ It is not possible to take reasonable steps to cure the breach or end the violation, as applicable.
	• If terminating the contract is not feasible, report the problem to the Secretary of HHS.
		• Have standards and thresholds for termination of the contract been included in the contract?

5. Government Entities May Satisfy Business Associate Contract Requirements through Other Arrangements
 	
Implementation Specification (Required)
	• If the covered entity and business associate are both governmental entities, consult § 164.314 (a)(2)(ii) of the Security Rule.
	• *If both entities are governmental entities, the covered entity is in compliance with § 164.314 (a)(1) if:*
	   ○ *It executes a Memorandum of Understanding (MOU) with the business associate that contains terms that accomplish the objectives of § 164.314(a)(2)(i), or*
	   ○ *Other law (including regulations adopted by the covered entity or its business associate) contains requirements applicable to the business associate that accomplish the objectives of § 164.314(a)(2)(i).*
		• Do the arrangements provide protections for EPHI equivalent to those provided by the organization's business associate contracts?
		• If termination of the MOU is not possible due to the nature of the relationship between the covered entity and the business associate, are other mechanisms for enforcement available, reasonable, and appropriate?

6. Other Arrangements for Covered Entities and Business Associates. Implementation Specification (Required)	• *If a business associate is required by law to perform a function or activity on behalf of a covered entity or to provide a service described in the definition of business associate as specified in §160.103 to a covered entity, the covered entity may permit the business associate to create, receive, maintain, or transmit electronic protected health information on its behalf to the extent necessary to comply with the legal mandate without meeting the requirements of § 164.314(a)(2)(i), provided that the covered entity attempts in good faith to obtain satisfactory assurances as required by § 164.314(a)(2)(ii)(A), and documents the attempt and the reasons that these assurances cannot be obtained.*	• Has the covered entity made a good faith attempt to obtain satisfactory assurances that the security standards required by this section are met? • Are attempts to obtain satisfactory assurances and the reasons assurances cannot be obtained documented? • Does the covered entity or its business associate have statutory obligations which require removal of the authorization of termination requirement?

An Introductory Resource Guide for Implementing the HIPAA Security Rule

Key Activities	Description	Sample Questions
	• The covered entity may omit from its other arrangements authorization of the termination of the contract by the covered entity, as required by § 164.314(a)(2)(i)(D), if such authorization is inconsistent with the statutory obligations of the covered entity or its business associate.	

An Introductory Resource Guide for Implementing the HIPAA Security Rule

4.20. Requirements for Group Health Plans (§ 164.314(b)(1))

HIPAA Standard: *Except when the only electronic protected health information disclosed to a plan sponsor is disclosed pursuant to § 164.504(f)(1)(ii) or (iii), or as authorized under § 164.508, a group health plan must ensure that its plan documents provide that the plan sponsor will reasonably and appropriately safeguard electronic protected health information created, received, maintained, or transmitted to or by the plan sponsor on behalf of the group health plan.*

Key Activities	Description	Sample Questions
1. Amend Plan Documents of Group Health Plan to Address Plan Sponsor's Security of EPHI Implementation Specification (Required)	• Amend plan documents to incorporate provisions to require the plan sponsor (e.g., an entity that sponsors a health plan) to implement administrative, technical, and physical safeguards that will reasonably and appropriately protect the confidentiality, integrity, and availability of EPHI that it creates, receives, maintains, or transmits on behalf of the group health plan.	• Does the plan sponsor fall under the exception described in the standard? • Do the plan documents require the plan sponsor to reasonably and appropriately safeguard EPHI?
2. Amend Plan Documents of Group Health Plan to Address Adequate Separation Implementation Specification (Required)	• Amend plan documents to ensure that the adequate separation between the group health plan and plan sponsor required by §164.504(f)(2)(iii) is supported by reasonable and appropriate security measures.	• Do plan documents address the obligation to keep EPHI secure with respect to the plan sponsor's employees, classes of employees, or other persons who will be given access to EPHI?
3. Amend Plan Documents of Group Health Plan to Address Security of EPHI Supplied to Plan Sponsors' Agents and Subcontractors Implementation Specification (Required)	• Amend plan documents to incorporate provisions to require the plan sponsor to ensure that any agent, including a subcontractor, to whom it provides EPHI agrees to implement reasonable and appropriate security measures to protect the EPHI.	• Do the plan documents of the group health plan address the issue of subcontractors and other agents of the plan sponsor implementing reasonable and appropriate security measures?
4. Amend Plan Documents of Group Health Plans to Address Reporting of Security Incidents Implementation Specification (Required)	• Amend plan documents to incorporate provisions to require the plan sponsor to report to the group health plan any security incident of which it becomes aware. • Establish specific policy for security incident reporting.[115] • Establish a reporting mechanism and a process for the plan sponsor to use in the event of a security incident.	• Is there a procedure in place for security incident reporting? • Are procedures in place for responding to security incidents?

---

[115] See Section 4.6, *HIPAA Standard: Security Incident Procedures.*

An Introductory Resource Guide for Implementing the HIPAA Security Rule

Policies and Procedures and Documentation Requirements

4.21. Policies and Procedures (§ 164.316(a))

HIPAA Standard: *Implement reasonable and appropriate policies and procedures to comply with the standards, implementation specifications, or other requirements of this subpart, taking into account those factors specified in § 164.306(b)(2)(i), (ii), (iii), and (iv). This standard is not to be construed to permit or excuse an action that violates any other standard, implementation specification, or other requirements of this subpart. A covered entity may change its policies and procedures at any time, provided that the changes are documented and are implemented in accordance with this subpart.*

Key Activities	Description	Sample Questions

1. Create and Deploy Policies and Procedures	• Implement reasonable and appropriate policies and procedures to comply with the standards, implementation specifications, and other requirements of the HIPAA Security Rule.
	• Periodically evaluate written policies and procedures to verify that:[116]
	  ○ Policies and procedures are sufficient to address the standards, implementation specifications, and other requirements of the HIPAA Security Rule.
	  ○ Policies and procedures accurately reflect the actual activities and practices exhibited by the covered entity, its staff, its systems, and its business associates.
		• Are reasonable and appropriate policies and procedures to comply with the standards, implementation specifications, and other requirements of the HIPAA Security Rule in place?
		• Are policies and procedures reasonable and appropriate given:
		  ○ the size, complexity, and capabilities of the covered entity;
		  ○ the covered entity's technical infrastructure, hardware, and software security capabilities;
		  ○ the costs for security measures; and
		  ○ the probability and criticality of potential risks to EPHI?
		  ○ Do procedures exist for periodically reevaluating the policies and procedures, updating them as necessary?[117]

2. Update Documentation of Policy and Procedures	• Change policies and procedures as is reasonable and appropriate, at any time, provided that the changes are documented and implemented in accordance with the requirements of the HIPAA Security Rule.	• Should HIPAA documentation be updated in response to periodic evaluations, following security incidents, and/or after acquisitions of new technology or new procedures? As policies and procedures are changed, are new versions made available and are workforce members appropriately trained?[118]

---

[116] See Section 4.8, *HIPAA Standard: Evaluation.*
[117] See Section 4.8, *HIPAA Standard: Evaluation.*
[118] See Section 4.22, *HIPAA Standard: Documentation* and Section 4.5, *HIPAA Standard: Security Awareness and Training.*

An Introductory Resource Guide for Implementing the HIPAA Security Rule

4.22. Documentation (§ 164.316(b)(1))

HIPAA Standard: *(i) Maintain the policies and procedures implemented to comply with this subpart in written (which may be electronic) form; and (ii) if an action, activity or assessment is required by this subpart to be documented, maintain a written (which may be electronic) record of the action, activity, or assessment.*

Key Activities	Description	Sample Questions
1. Draft, Maintain and Update Required Documentation	• Document the decisions concerning the management, operational, and technical controls selected to mitigate identified risks. • Written documentation may be incorporated into existing manuals, policies, and other documents, or may be created specifically for the purpose of demonstrating compliance with the HIPAA Security Rule.	• Are all required policies and procedures documented? • Should HIPAA Security Rule documentation be maintained by the individual responsible for HIPAA Security implementation? • Should HIPAA Security documentation updated in response to periodic evaluations, following security incidents, and/or after acquisitions of new technology or new procedures?
2. Retain Documentation for at Least Six Years Implementation Specifications (Required)	• *Retain required documentation of policies, procedures, actions, activities or assessments required by the HIPAA Security Rule for six years from the date of its creation or the date when it last was in effect, whichever is later.*	• Have documentation retention requirements under HIPAA been aligned with the organization's other data retention policies?
3. Assure that Documentation is Available to those Responsible for Implementation Implementation Specification (Required)	• *Make documentation available to those persons responsible for implementing the procedures to which the documentation pertains.*	• Is the location of documentation known to all staff that needs to access it? • Is availability of the documentation made known as part of education, training and awareness activities?[119]
4. Update Documentation as Required Implementation Specification (Required)	• *Review documentation periodically, and update as needed, in response to environmental or operational changes affecting the security of the EPHI.*	• Is there a version control procedure that allows verification of the timeliness of policies and procedures, if reasonable and appropriate? • Is there a process for soliciting input into updates of policies and procedures from staff, if reasonable and appropriate?

---

[119] See Section 4.5, *HIPAA Standard: Security Awareness and Training.*

Appendix A: Glossary

This appendix provides definitions for those terms used within this document that are defined specifically in the HIPAA Security Rule. Definitions for basic security terms used frequently in NIST publications, including this document, are centrally located in NIST Interagency Report 7298, *Glossary of Key Information Security Terms*. This glossary is available on http://csrc.nist.gov.

Administrative Safeguards [45 Code of Federal Regulations (C.F.R.) Sec. 164.304]	Administrative actions, and policies and procedures, to manage the selection, development, implementation, and maintenance of security measures to protect electronic protected health information and to manage the conduct of the covered entity's workforce in relation to the protection of that information.
Addressable [45 C.F.R. Sec. 164.306(d)(3)]	Describing 21 of the HIPAA Security Rule's 42 implementation specifications. To meet the addressable implementation specifications, a covered entity must (i) assess whether each implementation specification is a reasonable and appropriate safeguard in its environment, when analyzed with reference to the likely contribution to protecting the entity's electronic protected health information; and (ii) as applicable to the entity - (A) Implement the implementation specification if reasonable and appropriate; or (B) if implementing the implementation specification is not reasonable and appropriate—(1) document why it would not be reasonable and appropriate to implement the implementation specification; and (2) implement an equivalent alternative measure if reasonable and appropriate.
Affiliated Covered Entities [45 C.F.R. Sec. 164.105(b)]	Legally separate covered entities that are under common ownership or control and that have all designated themselves as a single affiliated covered entity for the purposes of the Privacy and Security Rule (more precisely, those parts of the Rules appearing at 45 CFR, Part 160, Subparts C and E).
Agency [FIPS 200; 44 U.S.C, Sec. 3502]	Any executive department, military department, government corporation, government-controlled corporation, or other establishment in the executive branch of the government (including the Executive Office of the President) or any independent regulatory agency, but does not include: 1) the General Accounting Office; 2) the Federal Election Commission; 3) the governments of the District of Columbia and of the territories and possessions of the United States and their various subdivisions; or 4) government-owned, contractor-operated facilities, including laboratories engaged in national defense research and production activities. Also referred to as Federal Agency.
Authentication	The corroboration that a person is the one claimed.

[45 C.F.R. Sec. 164.304]

Availability
[45 C.F.R. Sec. 164.304]

The property that data or information is accessible and usable upon demand by an authorized person.

Business Associate
[45 C.F.R. Sec. 160.103]

(1) Except as provided in paragraph (2) of this definition, "business associate" means, with respect to a covered entity, a person who:

(i) On behalf of such covered entity or of an organized healthcare arrangement (as defined at 45 C.F.R. Sec. 164.501) in which the covered entity participates, but other than in the capacity of a member of the workforce of such covered entity or arrangement, performs, or assists in the performance of:

(A) A function or activity involving the use or disclosure of individually identifiable health information, including claims processing or administration, data analysis, processing or administration, utilization review, quality assurance, billing, benefit management, practice management, and repricing; or

(B) Any other function or activity regulated by this subchapter; or

(ii) Provides, other than in the capacity of a member of the workforce of such covered entity, legal, actuarial, accounting, consulting, data aggregation (as defined in Sec. 164.501 of this subchapter), management, administrative, accreditation, or financial services to or for such covered entity, or to or for an organized healthcare arrangement in which the covered entity participates, where the provision of the service involves the disclosure of individually identifiable health information from such covered entity or arrangement, or from another business associate of such covered entity or arrangement, to the person.

(2) A covered entity participating in an organized healthcare arrangement that performs a function or activity as described by paragraph (1)(i) of this definition for or on behalf of such organized healthcare arrangement, or that provides a service as described in paragraph (1)(ii) of this definition to or for such organized healthcare arrangement, does not, simply through the performance of such function or activity or the provision of such service, become a business associate of other covered entities participating in such organized healthcare arrangement.

(3) A covered entity may be a business associate of another covered entity.

Confidentiality
[45 C.F.R. Sec. 164.304]

The property that data or information is not made available or disclosed to unauthorized persons or processes.

Covered Entities
[45 C.F.R. Sec.160.103]

Covered entity means: (1) A health plan. (2) A healthcare clearinghouse. (3) A healthcare provider who transmits any health information in electronic form in connection with a transaction covered by this subchapter. (4) Medicare

	Prescription Drug Card Sponsors.
Electronic Protected Health Information (electronic PHI, or EPHI) [45 C.F.R. Sec.160.103]	Information that comes within paragraphs (1)(i) or (1)(ii) of the definition of protected health information (see "protected health information").
Healthcare Clearinghouse [45 C.F.R. Sec.160.103]	A public or private entity, including a billing service, repricing company, community health management information system or community health information system, and "value-added" networks and switches, that does either of the following functions: (1) Processes or facilitates the processing of health information received from another entity in a nonstandard format or containing nonstandard data content into standard data elements or a standard transaction. (2) Receives a standard transaction from another entity and processes or facilitates the processing of health information into nonstandard format or nonstandard data content for the receiving entity.
Healthcare Provider [45 C.F.R. Sec. 160.103]	A provider of services (as defined in section 1861(u) of the Social Security Act, 42 U.S.C. 1395x(u)), a provider of medical or health services (as defined in section 1861(s) of the Social Security Act, 42 U.S.C. 1395x(s)), and any other person or organization who furnishes, bills, or is paid for healthcare in the normal course of business.
Health Information [45 C.F.R. Sec. 160.103]	Any information, whether oral or recorded in any form or medium, that: (1) Is created or received by a healthcare provider, health plan, public health authority, employer, life insurer, school or university, or healthcare clearinghouse; and (2) Relates to the past, present, or future physical or mental health or condition of an individual; the provision of healthcare to an individual; or the past, present, or future payment for the provision of healthcare to an individual
Health Plan [45 C.F.R. Sec.160.103]	(1) Health plan includes the following, singly or in combination: (i) A group health plan, as defined in this section. (ii) A health insurance issuer, as defined in this section. (iii) An HMO, as defined in this section. (iv) Part A or Part B of the Medicare program under title XVIII of the Social Security Act. (v) The Medicaid program under title XIX of the Social Security Act, 42 U.S.C. 1396, et seq. (vi) An issuer of a Medicare supplemental policy (as defined in section 1882(g)(1) of the Social Security Act, 42 U.S.C.

1395ss(g)(1)).

(vii) An issuer of a long-term care policy, excluding a nursing home fixed-indemnity policy.

(viii) An employee welfare benefit plan or any other arrangement that is established or maintained for the purpose of offering or providing health benefits to the employees of two or more employers.

(ix) The healthcare program for active military personnel under title 10 of the United States Code.

(x) The veterans' healthcare program under 38 U.S.C. chapter 17.

(xi) The Civilian Health and Medical Program of the Uniformed Services (CHAMPUS) (as defined in 10 U.S.C. 1072(4)).

(xii) The Indian Health Service program under the Indian Healthcare Improvement Act, 25 U.S.C. 1601, et seq.

(xiii) The Federal Employees Health Benefits Program under 5 U.S.C. 8902, et seq. (xiv) An approved State child health plan under title XXI of the Social Security Act, providing benefits for child health assistance that meet the requirements of section 2103 of the Social Security Act, 42 U.S.C. 1397, et seq.

(xv) The Medicare + Choice program under Part C of title XVIII of the Social Security Act, 42 U.S.C. 1395w-21 through 1395w-28.

(xvi) A high-risk pool that is a mechanism established under State law to provide health insurance coverage or comparable coverage to eligible individuals.

(xvii) Any other individual or group plan, or combination of individual or group plans, that provides or pays for the cost of medical care (as defined in section 2791(a)(2) of the PHS Social Security Act, 42 U.S.C. 300gg-91(a)(2)).

(2) Health plan excludes:

(i) Any policy, plan, or program to the extent that it provides, or pays for the cost of, excepted benefits that are listed in section 2791(c)(1) of the PHS Act, 42 U.S.C. 300gg-91(c)(1); and

(ii) A government-funded program (other than one listed in paragraph (1)(i)-(xvi) of this definition):

(A) Whose principal purpose is other than providing, or paying the cost of, healthcare; or

(B) Whose principal activity is:

(1) The direct provision of healthcare to persons; or

(2) The making of grants to fund the direct provision of healthcare to persons.

Hybrid Entity
[45 C.F.R. Sec.164.103]

A single legal entity:

(1) That is a covered entity;

(2) Whose business activities include both covered and non-covered functions; and

(3) That designates healthcare components in accordance with paragraph § 164.105(a)(2)(iii)(C).

Implementation Specification
[45 C.F.R. Sec. 160.103]

Specific requirements or instructions for implementing a standard.

Individually Identifiable Health Information (IIHI)
[45 C.F.R. Sec. 160.103]

Information that is a subset of health information, including demographic information collected from an individual, and:

(1) Is created or received by a healthcare provider, health plan, employer, or healthcare clearinghouse; and

(2) Relates to the past, present, or future physical or mental health or condition of an individual; the provision of healthcare to an individual; or the past, present, or future payment for the provision of healthcare to an individual; and

(i) That identifies the individual; or

(ii) With respect to which there is a reasonable basis to believe the information can be used to identify the individual.

Information System
[45 C.F.R. Sec. 164.304]

An interconnected set of information resources under the same direct management control that shares common functionality. A system normally includes hardware, software, information, data, applications, communications, and people.[120]

Integrity
[45 C.F.R. Sec. 164.304]

The property that data or information have not been altered or destroyed in an unauthorized manner.

Medicare Prescription Drug Card Sponsors

[Pub. L. 108-173]

A nongovernmental entity that offers an endorsed discount drug program under the Medicare Modernization Act.

Physical Safeguards
[45 C.F.R. Sec. 164.304]

Physical measures, policies, and procedures to protect a covered entity's electronic information systems and related buildings and equipment from natural and environmental hazards, and unauthorized intrusion.

Protected Health Information (PHI)

Individually identifiable health information:

(1) Except as provided in paragraph (2) of this definition, that

---

[120] FISMA defines "information system" as "a discrete set of information resources organized for the collection, processing, maintenance, use, sharing, dissemination, or disposition of information." 44 U.S.C., Sec. 3502.

[45 C.F.R., Sec. 160.103]   is:

     (i) Transmitted by electronic media;

     (ii) Maintained in electronic media; or

     (iii) Transmitted or maintained in any other form or medium. (2) Protected health information excludes individually identifiable health information in:

     (i) Education records covered by the Family Educational Rights and Privacy Act, as amended, 20 U.S.C. 1232g;

     (ii) Records described at 20 U.S.C. 1232g(a)(4)(B)(iv); and

     (iii) Employment records held by a covered entity in its role as employer.

Required
[45 C.F.R. Sec. 164.306(d)(2)]

As applied to an implementation specification (see implementation specification, above], indicating an implementation specification that a covered entity must implement. All implementation specifications are either required or addressable (see "addressable" above).

Security
[44 U.S.C., Sec. 3542]

Protecting information and information systems from unauthorized access, use, disclosure, disruption, modification, or destruction in order to provide—

     (A) integrity, which means guarding against improper information modification or destruction, and includes ensuring information non-repudiation and authenticity;

     (B) confidentiality, which means preserving authorized restrictions on access and disclosure, including means for protecting personal privacy and proprietary information; and

     (C) availability, which means ensuring timely and reliable access to and use of information.

Standard
[45 C.F.R., Sec. 160.103]

A rule, condition, or requirement: (1) Describing the following information for products, systems, services or practices: (i) Classification of components. (ii) Specification of materials, performance, or operations; or (iii) Delineation of procedures; or (2) With respect to the privacy of individually identifiable health information.

Technical Safeguards
[45 C.F.R., Sec. 164.304]

The technology and the policy and procedures for its use that protect electronic protected health information and control access to it.

User
[45 C.F.R., Sec. 164.304]

A person or entity with authorized access.

Appendix B: Acronyms

The appendix lists acronyms used within this document.

AC	Access Control (NIST SP 800-53 security control family)
AT	Awareness and Training (NIST SP 800-53 security control family)
AU	Audit and Accountability (NIST SP 800-53 security control family)
BAC	Business Associate Contract
CA	Certification, Accreditation, and Security Assessments (NIST SP 800-53 security control family)
C&A	Certification and Accreditation
CFR	Code of Federal Regulations
CIO	Chief Information Officer
CM	Configuration Management (NIST SP 800-53 security control family)
CMS	Centers for Medicare and Medicaid Services
CP	Contingency Planning (NIST SP 800-53 security control family)
CSD	Computer Security Division
DHHS	Department of Health and Human Services
EPHI	Electronic Protected Health Information
FISMA	Federal Information Security Management Act
FIPS	Federal Information Processing Standard
HHS	Department of Health and Human Services
HIPAA	Health Insurance Portability and Accountability Act
IA	Identification and Authentication (NIST SP 800-53 security control family)
ID	Identification
IR	Incident Response (NIST SP 800-53 security control family)
ISP	Internet Service Provider
IT	Information Technology
ITL	Information Technology Laboratory
LAN	Local Area Network
MA	Maintenance (NIST SP 800-53 security control family)
MOU	Memorandum of Understanding
MP	Media Protection (NIST SP 800-53 security control family)
NIST	National Institute of Standards and Technology
NISTIR	NIST Interagency Report
OESS	Office of E-Health Standards and Services
OIG	Office of the Inspector General
OMB	Office of Management and Budget
PE	Physical and Environmental Protection (NIST SP 800-53 security control family)
PHI	Protected Health Information
PKI	Public Key Infrastructure
PL	Planning (NIST SP 800-53 security control family)
PS	Personnel Security (NIST SP 800-53 security control family)
RA	Risk Assessment (NIST SP 800-53 security control family)
SA	System and Services Acquisition (NIST SP 800-53 security control family)
SC	System and Communications Protection (NIST SP 800-53 security control family)
SI	System and Information Integrity (NIST SP 800-53 security control family)
SP	Special Publication
US-CERT	United States Computer Emergency Response Team
US	United States

Appendix C: References

Public Laws

Public Law 107-347, E-Government Act of 2002 (Title III: Federal Information Security Management Act [FISMA] of 2002), December 17, 2002.

Public Law 104-191, Health Insurance Portability and Accountability Act (HIPAA) of 1996, August 21, 1996.

Federal Regulations

Health Insurance Reform: Security Standards; Final Rule ("The HIPAA Security Rule"), 68 FR 8334, February 20, 2003.

Federal Information Processing Standards (FIPS) Publications

FIPS 140-2, *Security Requirements for Cryptographic Modules*, June 2001.

FIPS 199, *Standards for Security Categorization of Federal Information and Information Systems*, February 2004.

FIPS 200, *Minimum Security Requirements for Federal Information and Information Systems*, March 2006.

FIPS 201-1, *Personal Identity Verification (PIV) of Federal Employees and Contractors*, March 2006.

NIST Special Publications (SPs)

NIST SP 800-12, *An Introduction to Computer Security: The NIST Handbook*, October 1995.

NIST SP 800-14, *Generally Accepted Principles and Practices for Securing Information Technology Systems*, September 1996.

NIST SP 800-16, *Information Technology Security Training Requirements: A Role- And Performance-Based Model*, April 1998.

NIST SP 800-18 Revision 1, *Guide for Developing Security Plans for Information Technology Systems*, February 2006.

NIST SP 800-21, *Guideline for Implementing Cryptography in the Federal Government*, December 2005.

NIST SP 800-30, *Risk Management Guide for Information Technology Systems*, January 2002.

NIST SP 800-34, *Contingency Planning Guide for Information Technology Systems*, June 2002.

NIST SP 800-35, *Guide to Information Technology Security Services*, October 2003.

NIST 800-37, *DRAFT Guide for Security Authorization of Federal Information Systems: A Security Lifecycle Approach*, August 2008.

NIST SP 800-39, *DRAFT Managing Risk from Information Systems: An Organizational Perspective*, April 2008.

NIST SP 800-41, *Guidelines on Firewalls and Firewall Policy*, January 2002.

NIST SP 800-42, *Guideline on Network Security Testing*, October 2003.

NIST SP 800-45, Version 2, *Guidelines on Electronic Mail Security*, February 2007.

NIST SP 800-46, *Security for Telecommuting and Broadband Communications,* August 2002.

NIST SP 800-47, *Security Guide for Interconnecting Information Technology Systems,* September 2002.

NSIT SP 800-48, Revision 1, *Guide to Securing Legacy IEEE 802.11 Wireless Networks,* July 2008.

NIST SP 800-50, *Building an Information Technology Security Awareness and Training Program,* October 2003.

NIST SP 800-52, *Guidelines for the Selection and Use of Transport Layer Security (TLS) Implementations,* June 2005.

NIST SP 800-53, Revision 2, *Recommended Security Controls for Federal Information Systems,* December 2007.

NIST SP 800-53A, *Guide for Assessing the Security Controls in Federal Information Systems,* June 2008.

NIST SP 800-55, Revision 1, *Performance Measurement Guide for Information Security,* July 2008.

NIST SP 800-58, *Security Considerations for Voice Over IP Systems,* January 2005.

NIST SP 800-60, Revision 1, *Guide for Mapping Types of Information and Information Systems to Security Categories,* July 2008.

NIST SP 800-61, Revision 1, *Computer Security Incident Handling Guide,* March 2008.

NIST SP 800-63-1, *DRAFT Electronic Authentication Guide,* February 2008.

NIST SP 800-64 Revision 2, *Security Considerations in the Information Systems Development Life Cycle,* October 2008.

NIST SP 800-77, *Guide to IPsec VPNs,* December 2005.

NIST SP 800-81, *Secure Domain Name System (DNS) Deployment Guide,* May 2006.

NIST SP 800-83, *Guide to Malware Incident Prevention and Handling,* November 2005.

NIST SP 800-84, *Guide to Test, Training, and Exercise Programs for IT Plans and Capabilities,* September 2006.

NIST SP 800-86, *Guide to Integrating Forensic Techniques into Incident Response,* August 2006.

NIST SP 800-88, *Guidelines for Media Sanitization,* September 2006.

NIST SP 800-92, *Guide to Computer Security Log Management,* September 2006.

NIST SP 800-94, *Guide to Intrusion Detection and Prevention Systems (IDPS),* February 2007.

NIST SP 800-100, *Information Security Handbook: A Guide for Managers,* October 2006.

NIST SP 800-106, *DRAFT Randomized Hashing Digital Signatures,* July 2008.

NIST SP 800-107, *DRAFT Recommendation for Using Approved Hash Algorithms,* July 2008.

NIST SP 800-111, *Guide to Storage Encryption Technologies for End User Devices,* November 2007.

NIST SP 800-113, *Guide to SSL VPNs,* July 2008.

NIST SP 800-114, *User's Guide to Securing External Devices for Telework and Remote Access*, November 2007.

NIST SP 800-115, *Technical Guide to Information Security Testing*, November 2007.

NIST SP 800-124, *DRAFT Guidelines on Cell Phone and PDA Security*, July 2008.

NIST Interagency Reports (NISTIRs)

NISTIR 7298, *Glossary of Key Information Security Terms*, April 2006.

CMS HIPAA Security Series Publications

Security 101 for Covered Entities, March 2007.

Security Standards Administrative Safeguards, March 2007.

Security Standards Physical Safeguards, March 2007.

Security Standards Technical Safeguards, March 2007.

Security Standards Organizational Policies, March 2007.

Basics of Risk Analysis and Risk Management, March 2007.

HIPAA Security Guidance for Remote Use of and Access to Electronic Protected Health Information, December 2006

Web sites and Other Resources

NIST: Computer Security Resource Center (CSRC): http://csrc.nist.gov/

NIST: National Vulnerability Database (NVD): http://nvd.nist.gov/

Guide to NIST Information Security Documents:
http://csrc.nist.gov/publications/CSD_DocsGuide.pdf

Department of Health and Human Services (DHHS), Centers for Medicare and Medicaid Services (CMS), HIPAA Resources: http://www.cms.hhs.gov/hipaa/hipaa2.

Workgroup for Electronic Data Interchange (WEDI): http://www.wedi.org

Appendix D: Security Rule Standards and Implementation Specifications Crosswalk

Appendix D provides a catalog (see Table 4) of the HIPAA Security Rule standards and implementation specifications within the Administrative, Physical, and Technical Safeguards sections of the Security Rule. Additionally, this catalog crosswalks, or maps, those Security Rule standards and implementation specifications to NIST publications relevant to each Security Rule standard, and to applicable security controls detailed in NIST SP 800-53, *Recommended Security Controls for Federal Information Systems*. Readers may draw upon these NIST publications and security controls for consideration in implementing the Security Rule.

The catalog is organized according to the categorization of standards within each of the safeguards sections in the Security Rule. Table 3 provides an overview of the catalog content.

Table 3. Overview of Catalog Content

Column Headers	Description
Section of HIPAA Security Rule	Indicates the regulatory citation to the appropriate section of the Security Rule where the standard and implementation specification can be found.
Standards	Lists the Security Rule Standards.
Implementation Specifications	Lists the implementation specifications associated with the standard, if any exist, and designates the specification as required or addressable. (*R = Required, A = Addressable*)
NIST SP 800-53 Security Controls Mapping	Provides a listing of NIST SP 800-53 security controls that may provide value when implementing the particular standards and implementation specifications. For full security control specifications, refer to NIST SP 800-53, which can be found online at http://csrc.nist.gov.
NIST Publications Crosswalk	Provides a listing of NIST publications that support each particular standard. Publications are listed by publication number. For the full publication title, refer to *Appendix C: References* within this document, or to the *Guide to NIST Information Security Documents* located on the NIST Computer Security Resource Center (CSRC) Web site at http://csrc.nist.gov.

The mapping of SP 800-53 security controls to Security Rule standards and implementation specifications is of particular importance because it allows for the traceability of legislative and regulatory directives, such as HIPAA and FISMA, to underlying technical security configurations. This mapping can also enable standards-based measurement and monitoring of technical security safeguards and computer security configurations; facilitate compliance management by automating portions of compliance demonstration and reporting; and reduce the chance of misinterpretation between auditors and operations teams.

To accomplish this automation, NIST has defined, and maintains, the Security Content Automation Protocol (SCAP),[121] a suite of selected and integrated open standards that enable standards-based communication of vulnerability data, customizing and managing configuration baselines for various IT products, assessing information systems and reporting compliance status, using standard measures to weigh and aggregate potential vulnerability impact, and remediating identified vulnerabilities.

---

[121] More information on the Security Content Automation Protocol (SCAP) is available on the National Vulnerability Web site, http://nvd.nist.gov.

Table 4. HIPAA Standards and Implementation Specifications Catalog

Section of HIPAA Security Rule	HIPAA Security Rule Standards	Implementation Specifications	NIST SP 800-53 Security Controls Mapping	NIST Publications Crosswalk
		Administrative Safeguards		
164.308(a)(1)(i)	Security Management Process: Implement policies and procedures to prevent, detect, contain, and correct security violations.		RA-1	FIPS 199 NIST SP 800-14 NIST SP 800-18 NIST SP 800-30 NIST SP 800-37 NIST Draft SP 800-39 NIST SP 800-42 NIST SP 800-53 NIST SP 800-55 NIST SP 800-60 NIST SP 800-84 NIST SP 800-92 NIST SP 800-100
164.308(a)(1)(ii)(A)		Risk Analysis (R): Conduct an accurate and thorough assessment of the potential risks and vulnerabilities to the confidentiality, integrity, and availability of electronic protected health information held by the covered entity.	RA-2, RA-3, RA-4	
164.308(a)(1)(ii)(B)		Risk Management (R): Implement security measures sufficient to reduce risks and vulnerabilities to a reasonable and appropriate level to comply with Section 164.306(a).	RA-2, RA-3, RA-4, PL-6	
164.308(a)(1)(ii)(C)		Sanction Policy (R): Apply appropriate sanctions against workforce members who fail to comply with the security policies and procedures of the covered entity.	PS-8	
164.308(a)(1)(ii)(D)		Information System Activity Review (R): Implement procedures to regularly review records of information system activity, such as audit logs, access reports, and security incident tracking reports.	AU-6, AU-7, CA-7, IR-5, IR-6, SI-4	
164.308(a)(2)	Assigned Security Responsibility: Identify the security official who is responsible for the development and implementation of the policies and procedures required by this subpart for the entity.		CA-4, CA-6	NIST SP 800-12 NIST SP 800-14 NIST SP 800 37 NIST SP 800-53 NIST SP 800-53A NIST SP 800-100

Section of HIPAA Security Rule	HIPAA Security Rule Standards	Implementation Specifications	NIST SP 800-53 Security Controls Mapping	NIST Publications Crosswalk
164.308(a)(3)(i)	Workforce Security: Implement policies and procedures to ensure that all members of its workforce have appropriate access to electronic protected health information, as provided under paragraph (a)(4) of this section, and to prevent those workforce members who do not have access under paragraph (a)(4) of this section from obtaining access to electronic protected health information.		AC-1, AC-5, AC-6	NIST SP 800-12 NIST SP 800-14 NIST SP 800-53
164.308(a)(3)(ii)(A)		Authorization and/or Supervision (A): Implement procedures for the authorization and/or supervision of workforce members who work with electronic protected health information or in locations where it might be accessed.	AC-1, AC-3, AC-4, AC-13, MA-5, MP-2, PS-1, PS-6, PS-7	
164.308(a)(3)(ii)(B)		Workforce Clearance Procedure (A): Implement procedures to determine that the access of a workforce member to electronic protected health information is appropriate.	AC-2, PS-1, PS-2, PS-3, PS-6	
164.308(a)(3)(ii)(C)		Termination Procedure (A): Implement procedures for terminating access to electronic protected health information when the employment of a workforce member ends or as required by determinations made as specified in paragraph (a)(3)(ii)(B) of this section.	PS-1, PS-4, PS-5	
164.308(a)(4)(i)	Information Access Management: Implement policies and procedures for authorizing access to electronic protected health information that are consistent with the applicable requirements of subpart E of this part.		AC-1, AC-2, AC-5, AC-6, AC-13	NIST SP 800-12 NIST SP 800-14 NIST SP 800-18 NIST SP 800-53 NIST SP 800-63

Section of HIPAA Security Rule	HIPAA Security Rule Standards	Implementation Specifications	NIST SP 800-53 Security Controls Mapping	NIST Publications Crosswalk
164.308(a)(4)(ii)(A)		Isolating Healthcare Clearinghouse Functions (R): If a healthcare clearinghouse is part of a larger organization, the clearinghouse must implement policies and procedures that protect the electronic protected health information of the clearinghouse from unauthorized access by the larger organization.	AC-5, AC-6	NIST SP 800-100
164.308(a)(4)(ii)(B)		Access Authorization (A): Implement policies and procedures for granting access to electronic protected health information, for example, through access to a workstation, transaction, program, process, or other mechanism.	AC-1, AC-2, AC-3, AC-4, AC-13, PS-6, PS-7	
164.308(a)(4)(ii)(C)		Access Establishment and Modification (A): Implement policies and procedures that, based upon the entity's access authorization policies, establish, document, review, and modify a user's right of access to a workstation, transaction, program, or process.	AC-1, AC-2, AC-3	
164.308(a)(5)(i)	Security Awareness and Training: Implement a security awareness and training program for all members of its workforce (including management).		AT-1, AT-2, AT-3, AT-4, AT-5	NIST SP 800-12 NIST SP 800-14 NIST SP 800-16 NIST SP 800-50 NIST SP 800-61 NIST SP 800-83
164.308(a)(5)(ii)(A)		Security Reminders (A): Periodic security updates.	AT-2, AT-5, SI-5	
164.308(a)(5)(ii)(B)		Protection from Malicious Software (A): Procedures for guarding against, detecting, and reporting malicious software.	AT-2, SI-3, SI-4, SI-8	
164.308(a)(5)(ii)(C)		Log-in Monitoring (A): Procedures for monitoring log-in attempts and reporting discrepancies.	AC-2, AC-13, AU-2, AU-6	
164.308(a)(5)(ii)(D)		Password Management (A): Procedures for creating, changing, and safeguarding passwords.	IA-2, IA-4, IA-5, IA-6, IA-7	

Section of HIPAA Security Rule	HIPAA Security Rule Standards	Implementation Specifications	NIST SP 800-53 Security Controls Mapping	NIST Publications Crosswalk
164.308(a)(6)(i)	Security Incident Procedures: Implement policies and procedures to address security incidents.		IR-1, IR-2, IR-3	NIST SP 800-12 NIST SP 800-14 NIST SP 800-61 NIST SP 800-83 NIST SP 800-86 NIST SP 800-94
164.308(a)(6)(ii)		Response and Reporting (R): Identify and respond to suspected or known security incidents; mitigate, to the extent practicable, harmful effects of security incidents that are known to the covered entity; and document security incidents and their outcomes.	IR-4, IR-5, IR-6, IR-7	
164.308(a)(7)(i)	Contingency Plan: Establish (and implement as needed) policies and procedures for responding to an emergency or other occurrence (for example, fire, vandalism, system failure, and natural disaster) that damages systems that contain electronic protected health information.		CP-1	FIPS 199 NIST SP 800-12 NIST SP 800-14 NIST SP 800-18 NIST SP 800-30 NIST SP 800-34 NIST SP 800-60 NIST SP 800-84
164.308(a)(7)(ii)(A)		Data Backup Plan (R): Establish and implement procedures to create and maintain retrievable exact copies of electronic protected health information.	CP-9	
164.308(a)(7)(ii)(B)		Disaster Recovery Plan (R): Establish (and implement as needed) procedures to restore any loss of data.	CP-2, CP-6, CP-7, CP-8, CP-9, CP-10	
164.308(a)(7)(ii)(C)		Emergency Mode Operation Plan (R): Establish (and implement as needed) procedures to enable continuation of critical business processes for protection of the security of electronic protected health information while operating in emergency mode.	CP-2, CP-10	

Section of HIPAA Security Rule	HIPAA Security Rule Standards	Implementation Specifications	NIST SP 800-53 Security Controls Mapping	NIST Publications Crosswalk
164.308(a)(7)(ii)(D)		Testing and Revision Procedure (A): Implement procedures for periodic testing and revision of contingency plans.	CP-3, CP-4, CP-5	
164.308(a)(7)(ii)(E)		Applications and Data Criticality Analysis (A): Assess the relative criticality of specific applications and data in support of other contingency plan components.	RA-2, CP-2	
164.308(a)(8)	Evaluation: Perform a periodic technical and nontechnical evaluation, based initially upon the standards implemented under this rule and subsequently, in response to environmental or operational changes affecting the security of electronic protected health information that establishes the extent to which an entity's security policies and procedures meet the requirements of this subpart.		CA-1, CA-2, CA-4, CA-6, CA-7	NIST SP 800-12 NIST SP 800-14 NIST SP 800-37 NIST SP 800-42 NIST SP 800-53A NIST SP 800-55 NIST SP 800-84 NIST SP 800-115
164.308(b)(1)	Business Associate Contracts and Other Arrangements: A covered entity, in accordance with § 164.306, may permit a business associate to create, receive, maintain, or transmit electronic protected health information on the covered entity's behalf only if the covered entity obtains satisfactory assurances, in accordance with Sec. 164.314(a), that the business associate will appropriately safeguard the information.		CA-3, PS-7, SA-9	NIST SP 800-12 NIST SP 800-14 NIST SP 800-37 NIST SP 800-47 NIST SP 800-100

Section of HIPAA Security Rule	HIPAA Security Rule Standards	Implementation Specifications	NIST SP 800-53 Security Controls Mapping	NIST Publications Crosswalk
164.308(b)(4)		Written Contract or Other Arrangement (R): Document the satisfactory assurances required by paragraph (b)(1) of this section through a written contract or other arrangement with the business associate that meets the applicable requirements of § 164.314(a).	CA-3, SA-9	
Physical Safeguards				
164.310(a)(1)	Facility Access Controls: Implement policies and procedures to limit physical access to its electronic information systems and the facility or facilities in which they are housed, while ensuring that properly authorized access is allowed.		PE-1, PE-2, PE-3, PE-4, PE-5	NIST SP 800-12 NIST SP 800-14 NIST SP 800-18 NIST SP 800-30 NIST SP 800-34 NIST SP 800-53
164.310(a)(2)(i)		Contingency Operations (A): Establish (and implement as needed) procedures that allow facility access in support of restoration of lost data under the disaster recovery plan and emergency mode operations plan in the event of an emergency.	CP-2, CP-6, CP-7, PE-17	
164.310(a)(2)(ii)		Facility Security Plan (A): Implement policies and procedures to safeguard the facility and the equipment therein from unauthorized physical access, tampering, and theft.	PE-1, PL-2, PL-6	
164.310(a)(2)(iii)		Access Control and Validation Procedures (A): Implement procedures to control and validate a person's access to facilities based on their role or function, including visitor control, and control of access to software programs for testing and revision.	AC-3, PE-1, PE-2, PE-3, PE-6, PE-7, PE-8	

Section of HIPAA Security Rule	HIPAA Security Rule Standards	Implementation Specifications	NIST SP 800-53 Security Controls Mapping	NIST Publications Crosswalk
164.310(a)(2)(iv)		Maintenance Records (A): Implement policies and procedures to document repairs and modifications to the physical components of a facility which are related to security (for example, hardware, walls, doors, and locks).	MA-1[122], MA-2, MA-6	
164.310(b)	Workstation Use: Implement policies and procedures that specify the proper functions to be performed, the manner in which those functions are to be performed, and the physical attributes of the surroundings of a specific workstation or class of workstation that can access electronic protected health information.		AC-3, AC-4, AC-11, AC-12, AC-15, AC-16, AC-17, AC-19, PE-3, PE-5, PS-6	NIST SP 800-12 NIST SP 800-14 NIST SP 800-53
164.310(c)	Workstation Security: Implement physical safeguards for all workstations that access electronic protected health information to restrict access to authorized users.		MP-2, MP-3, MP-4, PE-3, PE-4, PE-5, PE-18	NIST SP 800-12 NIST SP 800-14 NIST SP 800-53
164.310(d)(1)	Device and Media Controls: Implement policies and procedures that govern the receipt and removal of hardware and electronic media that contain electronic protected health information into and out of a facility, and the movement of these items within the facility.		CM-8, MP-1, MP-2, MP-3, MP-4, MP-5, MP-6	NIST SP 800-12 NIST SP 800-14 NIST SP 800-34 NIST SP 800-53 NIST SP 800-88

---

[122] In NIST SP 800-53, the Maintenance security control family discusses maintenance activities relating to information systems. The same principles, however, can be applied to facility maintenance.

Section of HIPAA Security Rule	HIPAA Security Rule Standards	Implementation Specifications	NIST SP 800-53 Security Controls Mapping	NIST Publications Crosswalk
164.310(d)(2)(i)		Disposal (R): Implement policies and procedures to address the final disposition of electronic protected health information and/or the hardware or electronic media on which it is stored.	MP-6	
164.310(d)(2)(ii)		Media Reuse (R): Implement procedures for removal of electronic protected health information from electronic media before the media are made available for reuse.	MP-6	
164.310(d)(2)(iii)		Accountability (A): Maintain a record of the movements of hardware and electronic media and any person responsible therefore.	CM-8, MP-5, PS-6	
164.310(d)(2)(iv)		Data Backup and Storage (A): Create a retrievable exact copy of electronic protected health information, when needed, before movement of equipment.	CP-9, MP-4	
Technical Safeguards				
164.312(a)(1)	Access Control: Implement technical policies and procedures for electronic information systems that maintain electronic protected health information to allow access only to those persons or software programs that have been granted access rights as specified in § 164.308(a)(4).		AC-1, AC-3, AC-5, AC-6	NIST SP 800-12 NIST SP 800-14 NIST SP 800-21 NIST SP 800-34 NIST SP 800-53 NIST SP 800-63 FIPS 140-2
164.312(a)(2)(i)		Unique User Identification (R): Assign a unique name and/or number for identifying and tracking user identity.	AC-2, AC-3, IA-2, IA-3, IA-4	
164.312(a)(2)(ii)		Emergency Access Procedure (R): Establish (and implement as needed) procedures for obtaining necessary electronic protected health information during an emergency.	AC-2, AC-3, CP-2	

Section of HIPAA Security Rule	HIPAA Security Rule Standards	Implementation Specifications	NIST SP 800-53 Security Controls Mapping	NIST Publications Crosswalk
164.312(a)(2)(iii)		Automatic Logoff (A): Implement electronic procedures that terminate an electronic session after a predetermined time of inactivity.	AC-11, AC-12	
164.312(a)(2)(iv)		Encryption and Decryption (A): Implement a mechanism to encrypt and decrypt electronic protected health information.	AC-3, SC-13	
164.312(b)	Audit Controls: Implement hardware, software, and/or procedural mechanisms that record and examine activity in information systems that contain or use electronic protected health information.		AU-1, AU-2, AU-3, AU-4, AU-6, AU-7	NIST SP 800-12 NIST SP 800-14 NIST SP 800-42 NIST SP 800-53 NIST SP 800-53A NIST SP 800-55 NIST SP 800-92 NIST SP 800-115
164.312(c)(1)	Integrity: Implement policies and procedures to protect electronic protected health information from improper alteration or destruction.		CP-9, MP-2, MP-5, SC-8, SI-1, SI-7	NIST SP 800-12 NIST SP 800-14 NIST SP 800-53 NIST Draft SP 800-106 NIST Draft SP 800-107
164.312(c)(2)		Mechanism to Authenticate Electronic Protected Health Information (A): Implement electronic mechanisms to corroborate that electronic protected health information has not been altered or destroyed in an unauthorized manner.	SC-8, SI-7	
164.312(d)	Person or Entity Authentication: Implement procedures to verify that a person or entity seeking access to electronic protected health information is the one claimed.		IA-2, IA-3, IA-4	FIPS 201 NIST SP 800-12 NIST SP 800-14 NIST SP 800-53 NIST SP 800-63

Section of HIPAA Security Rule	HIPAA Security Rule Standards	Implementation Specifications	NIST SP 800-53 Security Controls Mapping	NIST Publications Crosswalk
164.312(e)(1)	Transmission Security: Implement technical security measures to guard against unauthorized access to electronic protected health information that is being transmitted over an electronic communications network.		SC-9	FIPS 140-2 NIST SP 800-12 NIST SP 800-14 NIST SP 800-21 NIST SP 800-24 NIST SP 800-41 NIST SP 800-42 NIST SP 800-45 NIST SP 800-46 NIST SP 800-48 NIST SP 800-52 NIST SP 800-53 NIST SP 800-58 NIST SP 800-63 NIST SP 800-77 NIST SP 800-81 NIST SP 800-113
164.312(e)(2)(i)		Integrity Controls (A): Implement security measures to ensure that electronically transmitted electronic protected health information is not improperly modified without detection until disposed of.	SC-8, SI-7	
164.312(e)(2)(ii)		Encryption (A): Implement a mechanism to encrypt electronic protected health information whenever deemed appropriate.	SC-9, SC-12, SC-13	

Organizational

Section of HIPAA Security Rule	HIPAA Security Rule Standards	Implementation Specifications	NIST SP 800-53 Security Controls Mapping	NIST Publications Crosswalk
164.314(a)(1)	Business Associate Contracts or Other Arrangements: (i) The contract or other arrangement between the covered entity and its business associate required by § 164.308(b) must meet the requirements of paragraph (a)(2)(i) or (a)(2)(ii) of this section, as applicable. (ii) A covered entity is not in compliance with the standards in § 164.502(e) and paragraph (a) of this section if the covered entity knew of a pattern of an activity or practice of the business associate that constituted a material breach or violation of the business associate's obligation under the contract or other arrangement, unless the covered entity took reasonable steps to cure the breach or end the violation, as applicable, and, if such steps were unsuccessful—(A) Terminated the contract or arrangement, if feasible; or (B) If termination is not feasible, reported the problem to the Secretary.		PS-6, PS-7, SA-9	NIST SP 800-35 NIST Draft SP 800-39 NIST SP 800-47 NIST SP 800-64 NIST SP 800-100

Section of HIPAA Security Rule	HIPAA Security Rule Standards	Implementation Specifications	NIST SP 800-53 Security Controls Mapping	NIST Publications Crosswalk
164.314(a)(2)(i)		Business Associate Contracts (R): The contract between a covered entity and a business associate must provide that the business associate will– (A) Implement administrative, physical, and technical safeguards that reasonably and appropriately protect the confidentiality, integrity, and availability of the electronic protected health information that it creates, receives, maintains, or transmits on behalf of the covered entity as required by this subpart; (B) Ensure that any agent, including a subcontractor, to whom it provides such information agrees to implement reasonable and appropriate safeguards to protect it; (C) Report to the covered entity any security incident of which it becomes aware; (D) Authorize termination of the contract by the covered entity if the covered entity determines that the business associate has violated a material term of the contract.	IR-6, PS-6, PS-7, SA-4, SA-9	
164.314(a)(2)(ii)		Other Arrangements: When a covered entity and its business associate are both governmental entities, the covered entity is in compliance with paragraph (a)(1) of this section, if– (1) It enters into a memorandum of understanding with the business associate that contains terms that accomplish the objectives of paragraph (a)(2)(i) of this section; or (2) Other law (including regulations adopted by the covered entity or its business associate) contains requirements applicable to the business associate that accomplish the objectives of paragraph (a)(2)(i) of this section.	CA-3, PS-6, PS-7, SA-9	

Section of HIPAA Security Rule	HIPAA Security Rule Standards	Implementation Specifications	NIST SP 800-53 Security Controls Mapping	NIST Publications Crosswalk
164.314(b)(1)	Requirements for Group Health Plans: Except when the only electronic protected health information disclosed to a plan sponsor is disclosed pursuant to § 164.504(f)(1)(ii) or (iii), or as authorized under § 164.508, a group health plan must ensure that its plan documents provide that the plan sponsor will reasonably and appropriately safeguard electronic protected health information created, received, maintained, or transmitted to or by the plan sponsor on behalf of the group health plan.		Does not map	NIST SP 800-35 NIST Draft SP 800-39 NIST SP 800-47 NIST SP 800-61 NIST SP 800-64 NIST SP 800-100
164.314(b)(2)(i)		Group Heath Plan Implementation Specification (R): The plan documents of the group health plan must be amended to incorporate provisions to require the plan sponsor to-- (i) Implement administrative, physical, and technical safeguards that reasonably and appropriately protect the confidentiality, integrity, and availability of the electronic protected health information that it creates, receives, maintains, or transmits on behalf of the group health plan.	Does not map	
164.314(b)(2)(ii)		Group Heath Plan Implementation Specification (R): The plan documents of the group health plan must be amended to incorporate provisions to require the plan sponsor to-- (ii) Ensure that the adequate separation required by § 164.504(f)(2)(iii) is supported by reasonable and appropriate security measures.	Does not map	

Section of HIPAA Security Rule	HIPAA Security Rule Standards	Implementation Specifications	NIST SP 800-53 Security Controls Mapping	NIST Publications Crosswalk
164.314(b)(2)(iii)		Group Heath Plan Implementation Specification (R): The plan documents of the group health plan must be amended to incorporate provisions to require the plan sponsor to-- (iii) Ensure that any agent, including a subcontractor, to whom it provides this information, agrees to implement reasonable and appropriate security measures to protect the information.	Does not map	
164.314(b)(2)(iv)		Group Heath Plan Implementation Specification (R): The plan documents of the group health plan must be amended to incorporate provisions to require the plan sponsor to-- (iv) Report to the group health plan any security incident of which it becomes aware.	Does not map	
Policies and Procedure and Documentation Requirements				
164.316(a)	Policies and Procedures: Implement reasonable and appropriate policies and procedures to comply with the standards, implementation specifications, or other requirements of this subpart, taking into account those factors specified in § 164.306(b)(2)(i), (ii), (iii), and (iv). This standard is not to be construed to permit or excuse an action that violates any other standard, implementation specification, or other requirements of this subpart. A covered entity may change its policies and procedures at any time, provided that the changes are documented and are implemented in accordance with this subpart.		PL-1, PL-2, PL-3, RA-1, RA-3	NIST SP 800-12 NIST SP 800-14 NIST SP 800-100

Section of HIPAA Security Rule	HIPAA Security Rule Standards	Implementation Specifications	NIST SP 800-53 Security Controls Mapping	NIST Publications Crosswalk
164.316(b)(1)	Documentation: (i) Maintain the policies and procedures implemented to comply with this subpart in written (which may be electronic) form, and (ii) If an action, activity or assessment is required by this subpart to be documented, maintain a written (which may be electronic) record of the action, activity, or assessment.		PL-2	NIST SP 800-18 NIST SP 800-53 NIST SP 800-53A
164.316(b)(2)(i)		Time Limit (R): Retain the documentation required by paragraph (b)(1) of this section for six years from the date of its creation or the date when it last was in effect, whichever is later.	Does not map	
164.316(b)(2)(ii)		Availability (R): Make documentation available to those persons responsible for implementing the procedures to which the documentation pertains.	Does not map	
164.316(b)(2)(iii)		Updates (R): Review documentation periodically, and update as needed, in response to environmental or operational changes affecting the security of the electronic protected health information.	PL-3	

Appendix E: Risk Assessment Guidelines

This appendix incorporates risk assessment concepts and processes described in NIST SP 800-30 Revision 1, *Effective Use of Risk Assessments in Managing Enterprise Risk*, the NIST Risk Management Framework, and the *HIPAA Security Series: Basics of Risk Analysis and Risk Management*. It is intended to assist covered entities in identifying and mitigating risks to acceptable levels.

The purpose of a risk assessment is to identify conditions where EPHI could be disclosed without proper authorization, improperly modified, or made unavailable when needed. This information is then used to make risk management decisions on whether the HIPAA-required implementation specifications are sufficient or what additional addressable implementation specifications are needed to reduce risk to an acceptable level.

Key Terms Defined

When talking about risk, it is important that terminology be defined and clearly understood. This section defines important terms associated with risk assessment and management.

- *Risk* is the potential impact that a threat can have on the confidentiality, integrity, and availability on EPHI by exploiting a vulnerability.
- *Threats* are anything that can have a negative impact on EPHI. Threats are:
    - Intentional (e.g., malicious intent); or
    - Unintentional (e.g., misconfigured server, data entry error).
- *Threat sources* are:
    - Natural (e.g., floods, earthquakes, storms, tornados);
    - Human (e.g., intentional such as identity thieves, hackers, spyware authors; unintentional such as data entry error, accidental deletions); or
    - Environmental (e.g., power surges and spikes, hazmat contamination, environmental pollution).
- *Vulnerabilities* are a flaw or weakness in a system security procedure, design, implementation, or control that could be intentionally or unintentionally exercised by a threat.
- *Impact* is a negative quantitative and/or qualitative assessment of a vulnerability being exercised on the confidentiality, integrity, and availability of EPHI.

It can be easy to confuse vulnerabilities and threats. An organization may be vulnerable to damage from power spikes. The threats that could exploit this vulnerability may be overloaded circuits, faulty building wiring, dirty street power, or too much load on the local grid. It is important to separate these two terms in order to assist in proper security control selection. In this example, security controls could range from installing UPS systems, additional fuse boxes, or standby generators, or rewiring the office. These additional security controls may help to mitigate the vulnerability but not necessarily for each threat.

HIPAA Risk Assessment Requirements

Standard 164.308(a)(1)(i), *Security Management Process*, requires covered entities to:

Implement policies and procedures to prevent, detect, contain, and correct security violations.

The Security Management Process standard includes four required implementation specifications. Two of these specifications deal directly with risk analysis and risk management.

1. **Risk Analysis (R**[123]**)** – 164.308(a)(1)(ii)(A): Conduct an accurate and thorough assessment of the potential risks and vulnerabilities to the confidentiality, integrity, and availability of electronic protected health information held by the covered entity.

2. **Risk Management (R)** – 163.308(a)(1)(ii)(B): Implement security measures sufficient to reduce risks and vulnerabilities to a reasonable and appropriate level to comply with Section 164.306(a).

How to Conduct the Risk Assessment:

Risk assessments can be conducted using many different methodologies. There is no single methodology that will work for all organizations and all situations. The following steps represent key elements in a comprehensive risk assessment program, and provide an example of the risk assessment methodology described in NIST SP 800-30. It is expected that these steps will be customized to most effectively identify risk for an organization based on its own uniqueness. Even though these items are listed as steps, they are not prescriptive in the order that they should be conducted. Some steps can be conducted simultaneously rather than sequentially.

1. **Scope the Assessment.** The first step in assessing risk is to define the scope of the effort, resulting in a general characterization of the information system, its operating environment, and its boundary. To do this, it is necessary to identify where EPHI is created, received, maintained, processed, or transmitted.

    The scope of a risk assessment should include both the physical boundaries of a covered entity's location as well as a logical boundary covering the media containing EPHI, regardless of its location. Ensure that the risk assessment scope takes into consideration the remote work force and telecommuters, and removable media and portable computing devices (e.g., laptops, removable media, and backup media).

2. **Gather Information.** During this step, the covered entity should identify:
    - The conditions under which EPHI is created, received, maintained, processed, or transmitted by the covered entity; and

---

[123] "R" indicates a required implementation specification.

- The security controls currently being used to protect the EPHI.

This step is essential to ensure that vulnerabilities and threats are correctly identified. For example, an invalidated belief that a policy is being followed can miss a potential vulnerability, and not knowing about portable media containing EPHI can miss a threat to that environment. The level of effort needed to gather the necessary information depends heavily on the scope of the assessment and the size of the covered entity.

3. **Identify Realistic Threats.** Often performed simultaneously with step 4, *Identify Potential Vulnerabilities*, the goal of this step is to identify the potential threat sources and compile a threat statement listing potential threat-sources that are applicable to the covered entity and its operating environment. The listing of threat sources should include realistic and probable human and natural incidents that can have a negative impact on an organizations ability to protect EPHI. Threats can be easily identified by examining the environments where EPHI is being used.

Many external sources can be used for threat identification. Internet searches, vendor information, insurance data, and crime statistics are all viable sources of threat data. Examples of some common threat sources are listed in Table 5 below.

Table 5. Common Threat Sources

Type	Examples
Natural	Floods, earthquakes, tornados, landslides, avalanches, electrical storms, and other such events
Human	Events that are either enabled by or caused by human beings, such as unintentional acts (inadvertent data entry) or deliberate actions (network-based attacks, malicious software upload, and unauthorized access to confidential information)
Environmental	Long-term power failure, pollution, chemicals, liquid leak

4. **Identify Potential Vulnerabilities.** Often performed simultaneously with step 3, *Identify Realistic Threats*, the goal of this step is to develop a list of vulnerabilities (flaws or weaknesses) that could be exploited by potential threat sources. This list should focus on realistic technical and nontechnical areas where EPHI can be disclosed without proper authorization, improperly modified, or made unavailable when needed.

Covered entities should use internal and external sources to identify potential vulnerabilities. Internal sources may include previous risk assessments, vulnerability scan and system security test results, and audit reports. External sources may include Internet searches, vendor information, insurance data, and vulnerability databases such as the National Vulnerability Database (http://nvd.nist.gov). At the end of this appendix, a suggested (but not all-inclusive) source list is provided that organizations may wish to use to help in vulnerability identification.

5. **Assess Current Security Controls.** Often performed simultaneously with step 2, *Gather Information*, the purpose of this step is to determine if the implemented or planned security controls will minimize or eliminate risks to EPHI. A thorough understanding of the actual security controls in place for a covered entity will reduce the list of vulnerabilities, as well as the realistic probability, of a threat attacking (intentionally or unintentionally) EPHI.

   Covered entities should evaluate technical and nontechnical security controls at all places where EPHI is created, received, maintained, processed, or transmitted. This evaluation should determine whether the security measures implemented or planned are adequate to protect EPHI, and whether those measures required by the Security Rule are in place, configured, and used properly. The appropriateness and adequacy of security measures may vary depending on the structure, size, and geographical dispersion of the covered entity.

6. **Determine the Likelihood and the Impact of a Threat Exercising a Vulnerability.** The next major step in measuring the level of risk is to determine the likelihood and the adverse impact resulting from a threat successfully exploiting a vulnerability. This information can be obtained from existing organizational documentation, such as business impact and asset criticality assessments. A business impact assessment prioritizes the impact levels associated with the compromise of an organization's information assets based on a qualitative or quantitative assessment of the sensitivity and criticality of those assets. An asset criticality assessment identifies and prioritizes the sensitive and critical organization information assets (e.g., hardware, software, systems, services, and related technology assets) that support the organization's critical missions.

   If these organizational documents do not exist, the system and data sensitivity can be determined based on the level of protection required to maintain the EPHI's confidentiality, integrity, and availability. The adverse impact of a security event can be described in terms of loss or degradation of any, or a combination of any, of the following three security objectives: integrity, availability, and confidentiality. Table 6 provides a brief description of each security objective and the consequence (or impact) of its not being met.

Table 6. Security Objectives and Impacts

Security Objective	Impacts
Loss of Confidentiality	System and data confidentiality refers to the protection of information from unauthorized disclosure. The impact of unauthorized disclosure of confidential information can range from the jeopardizing of national security to the disclosure of Privacy Act data. Unauthorized, unanticipated, or unintentional disclosure could result in loss of public confidence, embarrassment, or legal action against the organization.

Security Objective	Impacts
Loss of Integrity	System and data integrity refers to the requirement that information be protected from improper modification. Integrity is lost if unauthorized changes are made to the data or IT system by either intentional or accidental acts. If the loss of system or data integrity is not corrected, continued use of the contaminated system or corrupted data could result in inaccuracy, fraud, or erroneous decisions. Also, violation of integrity may be the first step in a successful attack against system availability or confidentiality. For all these reasons, loss of integrity reduces the assurance of an IT system.
Loss of Availability	If a mission-critical IT system is unavailable to its end users, the organization's mission may be affected. Loss of system functionality and operational effectiveness, for example, may result in loss of productive time, thus impeding the end users' performance of their functions in supporting the organization's mission.

Some tangible impacts can be measured quantitatively in terms of lost revenue, the cost of repairing the system, or the level of effort required to correct problems caused by a successful threat action. Other impacts, such as the loss of public confidence, the loss of credibility, or damage to an organization's interest, cannot be measured in specific units but can be qualified or described in terms of high, medium, and low impacts. Qualitative and quantitative methods can be used to measure the impact of a threat occurring

7. **Determine the Level of Risk.** The purpose of this step is to assess the level of risk to the IT system. The determination of risk takes into account the information gathered and determinations made during the previous steps. The level of risk is determined by analyzing the values assigned to the likelihood of threat occurrence and resulting impact of threat occurrence. The risk-level determination may be performed by assigning a risk level based on the average of the assigned likelihood and impact levels. A risk-level matrix, such as the sample depicted in Table 7, can be used to assist in determining risk levels.

Table 7. Sample Risk-Level Matrix

Threat Likelihood	Impact		
	Low	Moderate	High
High	Low	Moderate	High
Moderate	Low	Moderate	Moderate
Low	Low	Low	Low

8. **Recommend Security Controls.** During this step, security controls that could mitigate the identified risks, as appropriate to the organization's operations, are recommended. The goal of the recommended controls is to reduce the level of risk to the IT system and its data to an acceptable level. Security control recommendations provide input to the risk mitigation process, during which the recommended security controls are evaluated, prioritized, and implemented.

   It should be noted that not all possible recommended security controls can be implemented to reduce loss. To determine which ones are required and appropriate for a specific organization, a cost-benefit analysis should be conducted for the proposed recommended controls, to demonstrate that the costs of implementing the controls can be justified by the reduction in the level of risk. In addition to cost, organizations should consider the operational impact and feasibility of introducing the recommended security controls into the operating environment.

9. **Document the Risk Assessment Results.**

   Once the risk assessment has been completed (threat sources and vulnerabilities identified, risks assessed, and security controls recommended), the results of each step in the risk assessment should be documented. NIST SP 800-30 provides a sample risk assessment report outline that may prove useful to covered entities.

Risk Assessment Results Affect Risk Management

The results of a risk assessment play a significant role in executing an organization's risk management strategy. In the context of the HIPAA Security Rule, the security control baseline, which consists of the standards and required implementation specifications, should be viewed as the foundation or starting point in the selection of adequate security controls necessary to protect EPHI. In many cases, additional security controls or control enhancements will be needed to protect EPHI or to satisfy the requirements of applicable laws, policies, standards, or regulations.

The risk assessment provides important inputs to determine the sufficiency of the security control baseline. The risk assessment results, coupled with the security control baseline, should be used to identify which addressable implementation specifications should be implemented to adequately mitigate identified risks.

Risk Assessment Resources

The following resources may provide useful information to assist covered entities in performing risk assessment, analysis, and management activities, and demonstrate compliance with the Security Management Process standard and related implementation specifications:

- HIPAA Security Series, Basics of Risk Analysis and Risk Management, 6/2005: rev. 3/2007;
  http://www.cms.hhs.gov/EducationMaterials/Downloads/BasicsofRiskAnalysisandRiskManagement.pdf

- NIST SP 800-30, *Risk Management Guide for Information Technology Systems*; http://csrc.nist.gov/publications/nistpubs/800-30/sp800-30.pdf
- Department of Homeland Security (DHS) National Infrastructure Protection Plan; http://www.dhs.gov/xprevprot/programs/editorial_0827.shtm
- NIST National Vulnerability Database (NVD); http://nvd.nist.gov/
- US-CERT; http://www.us-cert.gov/index.html
- Carnegie Mellon CERT Coordination Center; http://www.cert.org/insider_threat/

Appendix F: Contingency Planning Guidelines

Information technology (IT) and automated information systems are vital elements in most business processes. Because these IT resources are so essential to an organization's success, it is critical that the services provided by these systems are able to operate effectively without excessive interruption. Contingency planning supports this requirement by establishing thorough plans and procedures and technical measures that can enable a system to be recovered quickly and effectively following a service disruption or disaster. Interim measures may include the relocation of IT systems and operations to an alternate site, the recovery of IT functions using alternate equipment, or the performance of IT functions using manual methods.

IT systems are vulnerable to a variety of disruptions, ranging from mild (e.g., short-term power outage, disk drive failure) to severe (e.g., equipment destruction, fire). Vulnerabilities may be minimized or eliminated through technical, management, or operational solutions as part of the organization's risk management effort. However, it is virtually impossible to completely eliminate all risks. Contingency planning is designed to mitigate the risk of system and service unavailability by focusing efficient and effective recovery solutions.

Within the context of HIPAA, the goal of contingency planning is to adequately protect EPHI during a contingency event, and to ensure that organizations have their EPHI available when it is needed.

This appendix, Contingency Planning Guidelines, will identify fundamental planning principles and practices to help personnel develop and maintain effective information system contingency plans. This section will be based on NIST Special Publication 800-34, *Contingency Planning Guide for Information Technology Systems*.

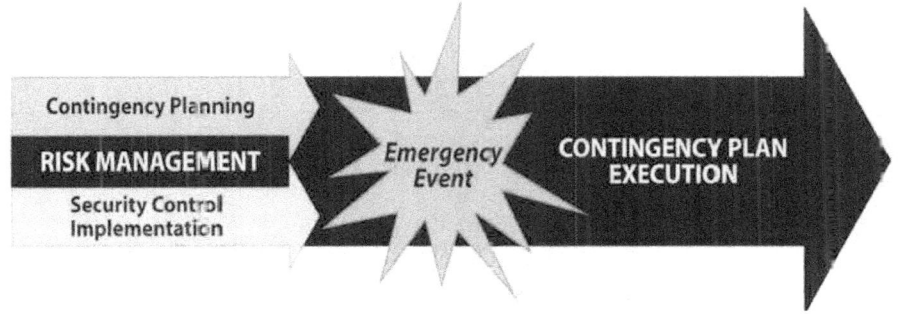

Contingency Planning Defined

IT contingency planning refers to a coordinated strategy involving plans, procedures, and technical measures that enable the recovery of IT systems, operations, and data after a disruption. Contingency planning generally includes one or more of the approaches to restore disrupted IT services:

- Restoring IT operations at an alternate location;
- Recovering IT operations using alternate equipment; and

- Performing some or all of the affected business processes using non-IT (manual) means (typically acceptable for only short-term disruptions).

Types of Contingency-Related Plans

IT contingency planning represents a broad scope of activities designed to sustain and recover critical IT services following an emergency. IT contingency planning fits into a much broader emergency preparedness environment that includes organizational and business process continuity and recovery planning. Ultimately, an organization would use a suite of plans to properly prepare response, recovery, and continuity activities for disruptions affecting the organization's IT systems, business processes, and the facility. Because there is an inherent relationship between an IT system and the business process it supports, there should be coordination between each plan during development and updates to ensure that recovery strategies and supporting resources neither negate each other nor duplicate efforts.

Table 8. Types of Contingency Plans

Type of Plan	Description	Scope
Contingency Plan (CP)	Management policy and procedures designed to maintain or restore business operations, including computer operations, possibly at an alternate location, in the event of emergencies, system failures, or disaster.	Addresses IT system disruptions; not typically business process-focused
Continuity of Operations Plan (COOP)	A predetermined set of instructions or procedures that describe how an organization's essential functions will be sustained for up to 30 days as a result of a disaster event before returning to normal operations.	Addresses the subset of an organization's missions that are deemed most critical; not typically IT-focused
Disaster Recovery Plan (DRP)	A written plan for processing critical applications in the event of a major hardware or software failure or destruction of facilities.	Limited to major disruptions with long-term effects; typically IT-focused

HIPAA Contingency Planning Requirements

Standard 164.308(a)(7), *Contingency Plan*, requires covered entities to:

Establish (and implement as needed) policies and procedures for responding to an emergency or other occurrence (for example, fire, vandalism, system failure, and natural disaster) that damages systems that contain electronic protected health information

The Contingency Plan standard includes five implementation specifications.

1. **Data Backup Plan (R)** – 164.308(a)(7)(ii)(A): Establish and implement procedures to create and maintain retrievable exact copies of electronic protected health information.

2. **Disaster Recovery Plan (R)** – 164.308(a)(7)(ii)(B): Establish (and implement as needed) procedures to restore any loss of data.

3. **Emergency Mode Operation Plan (R)** – 164.308(a)(7)(ii)(C): Establish (and implement as needed) procedures to enable continuation of critical business processes for protection of the security of electronic protected health information while operating in emergency mode.

4. **Testing and Revision Procedures (A)** – 164.308(a)(7)(ii)(D): Implement procedures for periodic testing and revision of contingency plans.

5. **Applications and Data Criticality Analysis (A)** – 164.308(a)(7)(ii)(E): Assess the relative criticality of specific applications and data in support of other contingency plan components.

IT Contingency Planning Process

To develop and maintain an effective IT contingency plan, organizations should consider using the approach discussed in NIST SP 800-34, *Contingency Planning Guide for Information Technology Systems*, which proposes a step-by-step contingency planning process, and provides an in-depth discussion of technical contingency planning considerations for specific types of information technology systems. A summary of this process is detailed below.

1. **Develop the Contingency Planning Policy Statement.** To be effective and to ensure that personnel fully understand the agency's contingency planning requirements, the contingency plan must be based on a clearly defined policy supported by organizational leadership. The contingency planning policy statement should define the organization's overall contingency objectives and establish the organizational framework and responsibilities for IT contingency planning. Key policy elements include:

    - Roles and responsibilities
    - Scope as applies to the type(s) of platform(s) and organization functions subject to contingency planning
    - Resource requirements
    - Training requirements
    - Exercise and testing, and plan maintenance schedules
    - Frequency of backups and storage of backup media.

2. **Conduct the Business Impact Analysis (BIA).** The BIA is a key step in the contingency planning process. The BIA enables the organization to fully characterize information system requirements, processes, and interdependencies and use this information to determine contingency requirements and priorities.

The purpose of the BIA is to correlate specific system components with the critical services that they provide and, based on that information, to characterize the consequences of a disruption to the system components. Key steps include identifying critical IT resources, disruption impacts and allowable outage times, and developing recovery priorities. Results from the BIA should be appropriately incorporated into the analysis and strategy development efforts for the organization's other continuity and recovery plans, including disaster recovery and emergency mode operations plans.

3. **Identify Preventive Controls.** In some cases, the outage impacts identified in the BIA may be mitigated or eliminated through preventive measures that deter, detect, and/or reduce impacts to the system. Where feasible and cost-effective, preventive methods are preferable to actions that may be necessary to recover the system after a disruption. Preventive controls should be documented in the contingency plan, and personnel associated with the system should be trained on how and when to use the controls.

A variety of preventive controls are available, depending on system type and configuration; however, some common measures are listed below:

- Appropriately sized uninterruptible power supplies (UPS) to provide short-term backup power to all system components (including environmental and safety controls)
- Gasoline- or diesel-powered generators to provide long-term backup power
- Air-conditioning systems with adequate excess capacity to permit failure of certain components, such as a compressor
- Fire suppression systems
- Fire and smoke detectors
- Water sensors in the computer room ceiling and floor
- Plastic tarps that may be unrolled over IT equipment to protect it from water damage
- Heat-resistant and waterproof containers for backup media and vital nonelectronic records
- Emergency master system shutdown switch
- Offsite storage of backup media, nonelectronic records, and system documentation
- Technical security controls, such as cryptographic key management and least-privilege access controls
- Frequent scheduled backups.

4. **Develop Recovery Strategies.** Recovery strategies provide a means to restore IT operations quickly and effectively following a service disruption. Strategies should address disruption impacts and allowable outage times identified in the BIA. Several alternatives should be considered when developing the strategy, including cost, allowable outage time, security, and integration with larger organization-level contingency plans.

   The selected recovery strategy should address the potential impacts identified in the BIA and should be integrated into the system architecture during the design and implementation phases of the system life cycle.

   The strategy should include a combination of methods that complement one another to provide recovery capability over the full spectrum of incidents, ranging from minor service disruption to a partial or total loss of primary system operations requiring operational resumption at another location. A wide variety of recovery approaches may be considered; the appropriate choice depends on the incident, type of system, and its operational requirements, including retention requirements. Specific recovery methods may include commercial contracts with cold, warm, or hot site vendors, mobile sites, mirrored sites, reciprocal agreements with internal or external organizations, and service-level agreements (SLAs) with the equipment vendors. In addition, high-availability technologies such as Redundant Arrays of Independent Disks (RAID), automatic fail-over, uninterruptible power supply (UPS), mirrored systems, and multisite data archiving systems should be considered when developing a system recovery strategy.

5. **Develop an IT Contingency Plan.** IT contingency plan development is a critical step in the process of implementing a comprehensive contingency planning program. The plan contains detailed roles, responsibilities, teams, and procedures associated with restoring an IT system following a disruption. The contingency plan should document technical capabilities designed to support contingency operations. Plans need to balance detail with flexibility; usually the more detailed the plan, the less scalable and versatile the approach.

   Following the approach described in NIST SP 800-34, the contingency plan comprises five main components: *Supporting Information, Notification and Activation, Recovery, Reconstitution,* and *Plan Appendices*. The first and last components provide essential information to ensure a comprehensive plan. The Notification and Activation, Recovery, and Reconstitution phases address specific actions that the organization should take following a system disruption or emergency.

   - The Supporting Information component includes an introduction and concept of operations section that provides essential background or contextual information that makes the contingency plan easier to understand, implement, and maintain. These details aid in understanding the applicability of the guidance, in making decisions on how to use the plan, and in providing information on where associated plans and information outside the scope of the plan may be found.

- The Notification and Activation Phase defines the initial actions taken once a system disruption or emergency has been detected or appears to be imminent. This phase includes activities to notify recovery personnel, assess system damage, and implement the plan. At the completion of the Notification and Activation Phase, recovery staff will be prepared to perform contingency measures to restore system functions on a temporary basis.

- The Recovery Phase begins after the contingency plan has been activated, damage assessment has been completed (if possible), personnel have been notified, and appropriate teams have been mobilized. Recovery phase activities focus on contingency measures to execute temporary IT processing capabilities, repair damage to the original system, and restore operational capabilities at the original or new facility. At the completion of the Recovery Phase, the IT system will be operational and performing the functions designated in the plan. Depending on the recovery strategies defined in the plan, these functions could include temporary manual processing, recovery and operation at an alternate system, or relocation and recovery at an alternate site. Teams with recovery responsibilities should understand and be able to perform these recovery strategies well enough that if the paper plan is unavailable during the initial stages of the event, they can still perform the necessary activities.

- In the Reconstitution Phase, recovery activities are terminated, and normal operations are transferred back to the organization's facility. If the original facility is unrecoverable, the activities in this phase can also be applied to preparing a new facility to support system processing requirements. Until the primary system is restored and tested, the contingency system should continue to be operated. The Reconstitution Phase should specify teams responsible for restoring or replacing both the site and the information system.

Contingency Plan Appendices should provide key details not contained in the main body of the plan. The appendices should reflect the specific technical, operational, and management contingency requirements of the information system and the larger organization. Appendices can include, but are not limited to, contact information for contingency planning team personnel; vendor contact information, including offsite storage and alternate site points of contact; standard operating procedures and checklists for system recovery or processes; equipment and system requirements lists of the hardware, software, firmware, and other resources required to support system operations; vendor agreements, reciprocal agreements with other organizations, and other vital records; description of, and directions to, the alternate site; and the BIA.

Plans should be formatted to provide quick and clear direction in the event those personnel unfamiliar with the plan or the systems are called on to perform recovery operations. Plans should be clear, concise, and easy to implement in an emergency. Where possible, checklists and step-by-step procedures should be used. A concise and well-formatted plan reduces the likelihood of creating an overly complex or confusing plan.

6. **Plan Testing, Training, and Exercises.** Plan testing is a critical element of a viable contingency capability. Testing enables plan deficiencies to be identified and addressed. Testing also helps evaluate the ability of the recovery staff to implement the plan quickly and effectively. Each IT contingency plan element should be tested to confirm the accuracy of individual recovery procedures and the overall effectiveness of the plan. The following areas should be addressed in a contingency test:

    - System recovery on an alternate platform from backup media
    - Coordination among recovery teams
    - Internal and external connectivity
    - System performance using alternate equipment
    - Restoration of normal operations
    - Notification procedures.

    Training for personnel with contingency plan responsibilities should complement testing. Training should be provided at least annually; new hires with plan responsibilities should receive training shortly after they are hired. Ultimately, contingency plan personnel should be trained to the extent that that they are able to execute their respective recovery procedures without aid of the actual document. This is an important goal in the event that paper or electronic versions of the plan are unavailable for the first few hours resulting from the extent of the disaster. Recovery personnel should be trained on the following plan elements:

    - Purpose of the plan
    - Cross-team coordination and communication
    - Reporting procedures
    - Security requirements
    - Team-specific processes (Notification/Activation, Recovery, and Reconstitution Phases)
    - Individual responsibilities (Notification/ Activation, Recovery, and Reconstitution Phases).

7. **Maintain the plan.** To be effective, the plan must be maintained in a ready state that accurately reflects system requirements, procedures, organizational structure, and policies. IT systems undergo frequent changes because of shifting business needs, technology upgrades, or new internal or external policies. Therefore, it is essential that the contingency plan be reviewed and updated regularly, as part of the organization's change management process, to ensure that new information is documented and contingency measures are revised if required. As a general rule,

Contingency Planning Resources

The following resources may provide useful information to assist covered entities in developing contingency planning strategies to adequately protect and recover access to EPHI during a contingency event, and demonstrate compliance with the Contingency Plan standard and implementation specifications:

- NIST Special Publication 800-34, *Contingency Planning Guide for Information Technology Systems*, http://csrc.nist.gov/publications/nistpubs/800-34/sp800-34.pdf
- HIPAA Security Series, Security Standards: Administrative Safeguards; http://www.cms.hhs.gov/EducationMaterials/Downloads/SecurityStandardsAdministrativeSafeguards.pdf

Appendix G: Sample Contingency Plan Template

This sample format provides a template for preparing an information technology (IT) contingency plan. The template is intended to be used as a guide and should be modified as necessary to meet the system's contingency requirements and comply with internal policies. Where practical, the guide provides instructions for completing specific sections. Text is added in certain sections; however, this information is intended only to suggest the type of information that may be found in that section. The text is not comprehensive and should be modified to meet specific organization and system considerations.

1. INTRODUCTION

1.1 PURPOSE

This {system name} Contingency Plan establishes procedures to recover the {system name} system following a disruption. The following objectives have been established for this plan:

- Maximize the effectiveness of contingency operations through an established plan that consists of the following phases:
    - **Notification/Activation phase** to detect and assess damage and to activate the plan;
    - **Recovery phase** to restore temporary IT operations and recover damage done to the original system; and
    - **Reconstitution phase** to restore IT system processing capabilities to normal operations.
- Identify the activities, resources, and procedures needed to carry out {system name} processing requirements during prolonged interruptions to normal operations.
- Assign responsibilities to designated {Organization name} personnel and provide guidance for recovering {system name} during prolonged periods of interruption to normal operations.
- Ensure coordination with other {Organization name} staff who will participate in the contingency planning strategies. Ensure coordination with external points of contact and vendors who will participate in the contingency planning strategies.

1.2 APPLICABILITY

The {system name} Contingency Plan applies to the functions, operations, and resources necessary to restore and resume {Organization name}'s {system name} operations as it is installed at its primary location: {Name, City, State}. The {system name} Contingency Plan applies to {Organization name} and all other persons associated with {system name} as identified under Section 2.3, Responsibilities.

1.3 SCOPE

1.3.1 Planning Principles

Various scenarios were considered to form a basis for the plan, and multiple assumptions were made. The applicability of the plan is predicated on two key principles:

- The {Organization name}'s facility in {City, State}, is inaccessible; therefore, {Organization name} is unable to perform {system name} processing for the organization.

- A valid contract exists with the alternate site that designates that site in {City, State}, as {Organization name}'s alternate operating facility.

    – {Organization name} will use the alternate site building and IT resources to recover {system name} functionality during an emergency situation that prevents access to the original facility.

    – The designated computer system at the alternate site has been configured to begin processing {system name} information.

    – The alternate site will be used to continue {system name} recovery and processing throughout the period of disruption, until the return to normal operations.

1.3.2 Assumptions

Based on these principles, the following assumptions were used when developing the IT Contingency Plan:

- The {system name} is inoperable at the {Organization name} computer center and cannot be recovered within {XX} hours.

- Key {system name} personnel have been identified and trained in their emergency response and recovery roles; they are available to activate the {system name} Contingency Plan.

- Preventive controls (e.g., generators, environmental controls, waterproof tarps, sprinkler systems, fire extinguishers, and fire department assistance) are fully operational at the time of the contingency event.

- Computer center equipment, including components supporting {system name}, are connected to an uninterruptible power supply (UPS) that provides {XX} minutes/hours of electricity during a power failure.

- {System name} hardware and software at the {Organization name} original site are unavailable for at least {XX} hours.

- Current backups of the application software and data are intact and available at the offsite storage facility.

- The equipment, connections, and capabilities required to operate {system name} are available at the alternate site in {City, State}.

- Service agreements are maintained with {system name} hardware, software, and communications providers to support the system recovery.

The {system name} Contingency Plan does not apply to the following situations:

- **Overall recovery and continuity of business operations.** The Business Resumption Plan (BRP) and Continuity of Operations Plan (COOP) are appended to the plan.
- **Emergency evacuation of personnel.** The Occupant Evacuation Plan (OEP) is appended to the plan.
- Any additional constraints should be added to this list.

1.4 REFERENCES/REQUIREMENTS

This {system name} Contingency Plan complies with the {Organization name}'s IT contingency planning policy as follows:

{Insert organization's contingency planning policy statement}

The {system name} Contingency Plan also complies with the following policies:

- Federal Information Security Management Act (FISMA) of 2002
- Health Insurance Portability and Accountability Act (HIPAA), 1996
- OMB Circular A-130, Management of Federal Information Resources, Appendix III, November 2000
- Federal Preparedness Circular (FPC) 65, Federal Executive Branch Continuity of Operations, July 1999
- PDD 63, Critical Infrastructure Protection, May 1998
- Federal Emergency Management Agency (FEMA), The Federal Response Plan (FRP), April 1999
- {Insert other applicable policies}

1.5 RECORD OF CHANGES

Modifications made to this plan are as follows:

Record of Changes			
Page No.	Change Comment	Date of Change	Signature

2. CONCEPT OF OPERATIONS

2.1 SYSTEM DESCRIPTION AND ARCHITECTURE

Provide a general description of system architecture and functionality. Indicate the operating environment, physical location, general location of users, and partnerships with external organizations/systems. Include information regarding any other technical considerations that are important for recovery purposes, such as backup procedures. Provide a diagram of the architecture, including security controls and telecommunications connections.

2.2 LINE OF SUCCESSION

The {organization name} sets forth an order of succession to ensure that decision-making authority for the {system name} Contingency Plan is uninterrupted. The Chief Information Officer (CIO), {organization name} is responsible for ensuring the safety of personnel and the execution of procedures documented within this {system name} Contingency Plan. If the CIO is unable to function as the overall authority or chooses to delegate this responsibility to a successor, the Deputy CIO shall function as that authority. Identify and describe line of succession as applicable.

2.3 RESPONSIBILITIES

The following teams have been developed and trained to respond to a contingency event affecting the IT system.

The Contingency Plan establishes several teams assigned to participate in recovering {system name} operations. Examples of teams that may be included are management team, application recovery team, operating system team, network operations team, site restoration/salvage team, procurement team, damage assessment team, and communications team. The system environment and the scope of the recovery effort will dictate which teams will be necessary to execute the plan.

- {Team name}
    - {*Describe each team, their responsibilities, leadership, and coordination with other applicable teams during a recovery operation. Do not detail specific procedures that will be used to execute these responsibilities. These procedures will be itemized in the appropriate phase sections.*}

The relationships of the teams involved in system recovery are illustrated in Figure {XX} below.

{*Insert hierarchical diagram of recovery teams. Show team names and leaders; do not include actual names of personnel.*}

3. NOTIFICATION AND ACTIVATION PHASE

This phase addresses the initial actions taken to detect and assess damage inflicted by a disruption to {system name}. Based on the assessment of the event, the plan may be activated by the Contingency Planning Coordinator.

In an emergency, the {Organization name}'s top priority is to preserve the health and safety of its staff before proceeding to the Notification and Activation procedures.

Notification

Contact information for key personnel is located in Appendix A. The notification sequence is listed below:

- The first responder is to notify the Contingency Planning Coordinator. All known information must be relayed to the Contingency Planning Coordinator.
- *{Insert further notification sequences specific to the organization and the system.}*

Upon notification, the following procedures are to be performed by their respective teams:

Damage Assessment Procedures:
{Detailed procedures should be outlined to include activities to determine the cause of the disruption; potential for additional disruption or damage; affected physical area and status of physical infrastructure; status of IT equipment functionality and inventory, including items that will need to be replaced; and estimated time to repair services to normal operations.}

- {team name}
    - Team Damage Assessment Procedures
- *{Insert additional team names and procedures as necessary}*

Activation

The Contingency Plan is to be activated if one or more of the following criteria are met:

1. {System name} will be unavailable for more than {XX} hours.
2. Facility is damaged and will be unavailable for more than {XX} hours.
3. Other criteria, as appropriate:

- If the plan is to be activated, the Contingency Planning Coordinator is to notify all Team Leaders and inform them of the details of the event and if relocation is required.
- Upon notification from the Contingency Planning Coordinator, Team Leaders are to notify their respective teams. Team members are to be informed of all applicable information and prepared to respond and relocate if necessary.
- The Contingency Planning Coordinator is to notify the offsite storage facility that a contingency event has been declared and to ship the necessary materials (as determined by damage assessment) to the alternate site.
- The Contingency Planning Coordinator is to notify the alternate site that a contingency event has been declared and to prepare the facility for the organization's arrival.
- The Contingency Planning Coordinator is to notify remaining personnel (via notification procedures) on the general status of the incident.

4. RECOVERY OPERATIONS

This section provides procedures for recovering the application at the alternate site, whereas other efforts are directed to repair damage to the original system and capabilities. The following procedures are for recovering the {system name} at the alternate site. Procedures are outlined per team required. Each procedure should be executed in the sequence it is presented to maintain efficient operations.

Recovery Goal. State the first recovery objective as determined by the Business Impact Assessment (BIA). For each team responsible for executing a function to meet this objective, state the team names and list their respective procedures.

- {team name}
  - Team Recovery Procedures
- *{Insert additional team names and procedures as necessary}*

Recovery Goal. State the remaining recovery objectives as determined by the BIA. For each team responsible for executing a function to meet this objective, state the team names and list their respective procedures.

- {team name}
  - Team Recovery Procedures
- *{Insert additional team names and procedures as necessary}*

5. RETURN TO NORMAL OPERATIONS

This section discusses activities necessary for restoring {system name} operations at the {Organization name}'s original or a new site. When the computer center at the original or the new site has been restored, {system name} operations at the alternate site must be transitioned back. The goal is to provide a seamless transition of operations from the alternate site to the computer center.

Original or New Site Restoration

Procedures should be outlined, per necessary team, to restore or replace the original site so that normal operations may be transferred. IT equipment and telecommunications connections should be tested.

- {team name}
  - Team Resumption Procedures
- *{Insert additional team names and procedures as necessary}*

5.1 CONCURRENT PROCESSING

Procedures should be outlined, per necessary team, to operate the system in coordination with the system at the original or the new site. These procedures should include testing the original or new system until it is functioning properly and ensuring that the contingency system is shut down gracefully.

- {team name}

– Team Concurrent Processing Procedures

- *{Insert additional team names and procedures as necessary}*

5.2 PLAN DEACTIVATION

Procedures should be outlined, per necessary team, to clean the alternate site of any equipment or other materials belonging to the organization, with a focus on handling sensitive information. Materials, equipment, and backup media should be properly packaged, labeled, and shipped to the appropriate location(s). Team members should be instructed to return to the original or the new site.

- {team name}

  – Team Deactivation Procedures

- *{Insert additional team names and procedures as necessary}*

6. PLAN APPENDICES

The appendices included should be based on system and plan requirements.

- *Personnel Contact List*
- *Vendor Contact List*
- *Equipment and Specifications*
- *Service-Level Agreements and Memorandums of Understanding*
- *IT Standard Operating Procedures*
- *Business Impact Analysis*
- *Related Contingency Plans*
- *Emergency Management Plan*
- *Occupant Evacuation Plan*
- *Continuity of Operations Plan.*

Appendix H: Resources for Secure Remote Use and Access

The HIPAA Security Rule requires all covered entities to protect the EPHI that they use or disclose to business associates, trading partners, or other entities. New technologies, such as remote access and removable media technologies, have significantly simplified the way in which data is transmitted throughout the healthcare industry and created tremendous opportunities for improvements and greater efficiency in the healthcare space. However, these technologies have also increased the risk of loss and unauthorized use and disclosure of this sensitive information. Sensitive information that is accessed by, stored on, or transmitted to or from a remote device needs to be protected so that malicious parties cannot access or alter it. An unauthorized release of sensitive information could damage the trust in an organization, jeopardize its mission, or harm individuals if their personal information has been released.

In December 2006, CMS issued a HIPAA security guidance document, *Remote Use of and Access to Electronic Protected Health Information*, to reinforce some of the ways a covered entity may protect EPHI when it is accessed or used outside of the organization's physical purview. It sets forth some strategies that may be reasonable and appropriate under the HIPAA Security Rule, for covered entities to follow (based upon their individual technological capabilities and operational needs), for offsite use of, or access to, EPHI. This guidance also places significant emphasis on the importance of risk analysis and risk management strategies, policies and procedures, and security awareness and training on the policies and procedures for safeguarding EPHI during its remote access, storage, and transmission.

NIST publications on remote access, storage, and transmission security technologies can be valuable resources to support secure remote use solutions. These publications seek to assist organizations in understanding particular technologies and to provide security considerations and practical, real-world recommendations for implementing and securing these technologies within an organization.

Special Publication 800-114, *User's Guide to Securing External Devices for Telework and Remote Access*, was developed to help teleworkers secure the external devices they use for telework, such as personally owned and third-party privately owned desktop and laptop computers and consumer devices (e.g., cell phones, personal digital assistants). The document focuses specifically on security for telework involving remote access to organizations' nonpublic computing resources by providing:

- Recommendations for securing telework computers' operating systems and applications, as well as home networks that the computers use;
- Basic recommendations for securing consumer devices used for telework;
- Advice on protecting the information stored on telework computers and removable media; and
- Tips on considering the security of a device owned by a third party before deciding whether it should be used for telework.

Special Publication 800-113, *Guide to SSL VPNs*, assists organizations in understanding SSL VPN technologies and in designing, implementing, configuring, securing, monitoring, and maintaining SSL VPN solutions. This publication intends to help organizations determine how best to deploy SSL VPNs within their specific network environments by:

- Describing SSL and how it fits within the context of layered network security;
- Presenting a phased approach to SSL VPN planning and implementation that can help in achieving successful SSL VPN deployments; and
- Comparing SSL VPN technology with IPsec VPNs and other VPN solutions.

Special Publication 800-77, *Guide to IPsec VPNs*, assists organizations in mitigating the risks associated with the transmission of sensitive information across networks by providing practical guidelines on implementing security services based on Internet Protocol Security (IPsec). This publication intends to help organizations determine how best to deploy IPsec VPNs within their specific network environments by:

- Discussing the need for, and types of, network layer security services and how IPsec addresses these services;
- Providing a phased approach to IPsec planning and implementation that can help in achieving successful IPsec deployments;
- Providing specific recommendations relating to configuring cryptography for IPsec;
- Using a case-based approach to show how IPsec can be used to solve common network security issues; and
- Discussing alternatives to IPsec and under what circumstances each may be appropriate.

Special Publication 800-52, *Guidelines for the Selection and Use of Transport Layer Security (TLS)*, provides guidelines on the selection and implementation of the TLS protocol while making effective use of Federal Information Processing Standards (FIPS)-approved cryptographic algorithms. TLS provides a mechanism to protect sensitive data during electronic dissemination across the Internet. This guideline:

- Describes the placement of security in each layer of the communications protocol stack, as defined by the OSI Seven Layer Model;
- Provides criteria for developing specific recommendations when selecting, installing and using transport layer security; and
- Discusses client implementation, server, and operational considerations.

Special Publication 800-111, *Guide to Storage Encryption Technologies for End User Devices*, assists organizations in understanding storage encryption technologies for end user devices and in planning, implementing, and maintaining storage encryption solutions. The types of end user devices addressed in this document are personal computers (desktops and laptops), consumer devices (e.g., personal digital assistants, smart phones), and removable storage media (e.g., USB flash drives, memory cards, external hard drives, writeable CDs and DVDs). This publication:

- Provides an overview of the basic concepts of storage encryption for end user devices;
- Provides guidelines on commonly used categories of storage encryption techniques (i.e., full disk, volume and virtual disk, and file/folder), and explains the types of protection they provide;
- Discusses important security elements of a storage encryption deployment, including cryptographic key management and authentication; and
- Examines several use cases which illustrate multiple ways to meet most storage encryption needs.

Draft Special Publication 800-124, *Guidelines on Cell Phone and PDA Security*, provides an overview of cell phone and personal digital assistant (PDA) devices in use today and offers insights for making informed information technology security decisions regarding their treatment. This publication:

- Presents an overview of handheld devices and discusses associated security threats and technology risks;
- Examines the security concerns associated with handheld devices; and
- Discusses user- and organization-oriented measures and safeguards available for mitigating the risks and threats.

All NIST publications are accessible on the public Computer Security Resource Center (CSRC) Web site at http://csrc.nist.gov.

Appendix I: Telework Security Considerations

Many people *telework*, which is the ability for an organization's employees and contractors to conduct work from locations other than the organization's facilities. Teleworkers use various devices, such as desktop and laptop computers, cell phones, and personal digital assistants (PDAs), to read and send email, access Web sites, review and edit documents, and perform many other tasks. Most teleworkers use *remote access*, which is the ability of an organization's users to access its nonpublic computing resources from locations other than the organization's facilities. Organizations have many options for providing remote access, including virtual private networks, remote system control, and individual application access (e.g., Web-based email).

This appendix provides considerations and tips for securing external devices used for telework and remote access. More detailed information on this topic is available in NIST SP 800-114, *User's Guide to Securing External Devices for Telework and Remote Access*.

Before teleworking, users should understand their organization's policies and requirements, as well as appropriate ways of protecting the organization's information that they may access.

Teleworkers should consult their organization's policies and requirements to provide adequate security to protect the organization's information. Sensitive information that is stored on, or sent to or from, external telework devices needs to be protected so that malicious parties can neither access nor alter it. An unauthorized release of sensitive information could damage the public's trust in an organization, jeopardize the mission of an organization, or harm individuals if their personal information has been released.

Teleworkers should ensure that all the devices on their wired and wireless home networks are properly secured, as well as the home networks themselves.

An important part of telework and remote access security is applying security measures to the personal computers (PCs) and consumer devices using the same wired and wireless home networks to which the telework device normally connects. If any of these other devices become infected with malware or are otherwise compromised, they could attack the telework device or eavesdrop on its communications. Teleworkers should also be cautious about allowing others to place devices on the teleworkers' home networks, in case one of these devices is compromised.

Teleworkers should apply security measures to the home networks to which their telework devices normally connect. One example of a security measure is using a broadband router or firewall appliance to prevent computers outside the home network from initiating communications with telework devices on the home network. Another example is ensuring that sensitive information transmitted over a wireless home network is adequately protected through strong encryption.

Teleworkers should consider the security state of a third-party device before using it for telework.

Teleworkers often want to perform remote access from third-party devices, such as checking email from a kiosk computer at a conference. However, teleworkers typically do not know if such devices have been secured properly or if they have been compromised. Consequently, a teleworker could use a third-party device infected with malware that steals information from users (e.g., passwords or email messages). Many organizations either forbid third-party devices to be used for remote access or permit only limited use, such as for Web-based email. Teleworkers should consider who is responsible for securing a third-party device and who can access the device before deciding whether or not to use it. Whenever possible, teleworkers should not use publicly accessible third-party devices for telework, and teleworkers should avoid using any third-party devices for performing sensitive functions or accessing sensitive information.

Secure a Telework PC

Teleworkers who use their own desktop or laptop PCs for telework should secure their operating systems and primary applications.

- Use a combination of security software, such as antivirus and antispyware software, personal firewalls, spam and Web content filtering, and popup blocking, to stop most attacks, particularly malware;

- Restrict who can use the PC by having a separate standard user account for each person, assigning a password to each user account, using the standard user accounts for daily use, and protecting user sessions from unauthorized physical access;

- Ensure that updates and patches are regularly applied to the operating system and primary applications, such as Web browsers, email clients, instant messaging clients, and security software;

- Disable unneeded networking features on the PC and configure wireless networking securely;

- Configure primary applications to filter content and stop other activity that is likely to be malicious;

- Install and use only known and trusted software;

- Configure remote access software based on the organization's requirements and recommendations; and

- Maintain the PC's security on an ongoing basis, such as changing passwords regularly and checking the status of security software periodically.

Secure consumer devices used for telework, such as cell phones, PDAs, and video game systems

A wide variety of consumer devices exists, and security features available for these devices also vary widely. Some devices offer only a few basic features, whereas others offer sophisticated features similar to those offered by PCs. This does not necessarily imply that more security features are better; in fact, many devices offer more security features because the capabilities they provide (e.g., wireless networking, instant messaging) make them more susceptible to attack than devices without these capabilities. General recommendations for securing telework devices are as follows:

- Limit access to the device, such as setting a personal identification number (PIN) or password and automatically locking a device after an idle period;
- Disable networking capabilities, such as Bluetooth, except when they are needed;
- Use additional security software, such as antivirus software and personal firewalls, if appropriate;
- Ensure that security updates, if available, are acquired and installed at least monthly, or more frequently; and
- Configure applications to support security (e.g., blocking activity that is likely to be malicious).

Secure Information

- Use physical security controls for telework devices and removable media. For example, an organization might require that laptops be physically secured using cable locks when used in hotels, conferences, and other locations where third parties could easily gain physical access to the devices. Organizations may also have physical security requirements for papers and other non-computer media that contain sensitive information and are taken outside the organization's facilities.
- Encrypt files stored on telework devices and removable media such as CDs and flash drives. This prevents attackers from readily gaining access to information in the files. Many options exist for protecting files, including encrypting individual files or folders, volumes, and hard drives. Generally, using an encryption method to protect files also requires the use of an authentication mechanism (e.g., password) to decrypt the files when needed.
- Ensure that information stored on telework devices is backed up. If something adverse happens to a device, such as a hardware, software, or power failure or a natural disaster, the information on the device will be lost unless it has been backed up to another device or removable media. Some organizations permit teleworkers to back up their local files to a centralized system (e.g., through VPN remote access), whereas other organizations recommend that their teleworkers perform local backups (e.g., burning CDs, copying files onto removable media). Teleworkers should perform backups, following their organizations' guidelines, and verify that the backups are valid and complete. It is important that backups on removable media be secured at least as well as the device that they backed up. For example, if a computer is stored in a locked room, then the media also should be in a secured location; if a computer stores its data encrypted, then the backups of that data should also be encrypted.
- Ensure that information is destroyed when it is no longer needed. For example, the organization's files should be removed from a computer scheduled to be retired or from a third-party computer that is temporarily used for remote access. Some remote access methods perform basic information cleanup, such as clearing

Web browser caches that might inadvertently hold sensitive information, but more extensive cleanup typically requires using a special utility, such as a disk-scrubbing program specifically designed to remove all traces of information from a device. Another example of information destruction is shredding telework papers containing sensitive information once the papers are no longer needed.

- Erase information from missing cell phones and PDAs. If a cell phone or PDA is lost or stolen, occasionally its contents can be erased remotely. This prevents an attacker from obtaining any information from the device. The availability of this service depends on the capabilities of the product and the company providing network services for the product.

Adequately protect remote access-specific authenticators

- Teleworkers need to ensure that they adequately protect their remote access-specific authenticators, such as passwords, personal identification numbers (PINs), and hardware tokens. Such authenticators should not be stored with the telework computer, nor should multiple authenticators be stored with each other (e.g., a password or PIN should not be written on the back of a hardware token).

Social Engineering

- Teleworkers should be aware of how to handle threats involving *social engineering*, which is a general term for attackers trying to trick people into revealing sensitive information or performing certain actions, such as downloading and executing files that appear to be benign but are actually malicious. For example, an attacker might approach a teleworker in a coffee shop and ask to use the computer for a minute or offer to help the teleworker with using the computer.

- Teleworkers should be wary of any requests they receive that could lead to a security breach or to the theft of a telework device.

Handling a Security Breach

- If a teleworker suspects that a security breach (including loss or theft of materials) has occurred involving a telework device, remote access communications, removable media, or other telework components, the teleworker should immediately follow the organization's policy and procedures for reporting the possible breach. This is particularly important if any of the affected telework components contain sensitive information such as EPHI, so that the potential impact of a security breach is minimized.